RESTORE
HEARING
NATURALLY

RESTORE HEARING NATURALLY

How to Use Your Inner Resources to Bring Back Full Hearing

ANTON STUCKI

Translated by Iren Izabella Toms

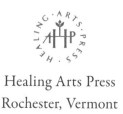

Healing Arts Press
Rochester, Vermont

Healing Arts Press
One Park Street
Rochester, Vermont 05767
www.HealingArtsPress.com

Healing Arts Press is a division of Inner Traditions International

Originally published in German under the title *Besser hören leichter leben* by AT Verlag
First U.S. edition published in 2020 by Healing Arts Press

The images on page 118 are from the book *Das sensible Chaos* by Theodor
Schwenk © Verlag Freies Geistesleben, Germany, and are used with permission.
This book is available in English under the title *Sensitive Chaos*.

Note to the reader: *This book is intended as an informational guide. The remedies,
approaches, and techniques described herein are meant to supplement, and not to be a
substitute for, professional medical care or treatment. They should not be used to treat
a serious ailment without prior consultation with a qualified health care professional.*

Cataloging-in-Publication Data for this title is available from the Library of Congress

ISBN 978-1-62055-893-5 (print)
ISBN 978-1-62055-894-2 (ebook)

Printed and bound in that United States by Versa Press, Inc.

10 9 8 7 6 5 4 3 2 1

Text design by Virginia Scott Bowman and layout by Debbie Glogover
This book was typeset in Garamond Premier Pro with Caecilia LT Std,
Futura Std, Gill Sans MT Pro, ITC Legacy Sans Std, and Metropolis used as
display fonts

To send correspondence to the author of this book, mail a first-class letter to the
author c/o Inner Traditions • Bear & Company, One Park Street, Rochester, VT
05767, and we will forward the communication, or contact the author directly at
www.Naturschallwandler.com.

A MANUAL TO RELEARN HOW TO HEAR WELL

These words are written
to encourage people
to go their own way
with their inherent powers of healing and regeneration—
to be whatever they want to be,
to do what lies in their hearts,
to understand what their minds need, to find peace,
and
to act rationally and with love.

Contents

Acknowledgments   xi

INTRODUCTION Rebuilding Our Connection to the World   1
The Three Pillars of the Method 5

How to Use This Book   8

PART 1

The Basics and the Basic Method
*Understanding Hearing Loss and
the Potential for Regeneration*

1 A Great Start Means Knowing Where
You're Going: Orientation to the Basics   12
Each Person Can Hear 15
The Process of Hearing 19
The Ability to Learn through Training 24
Relearning the Hearing Process 27
Physics and Acoustics 29
*Technical Implementation of the Naturschallwandler
(Natural Sound Transducer) 37*
EXERCISE: How Well Do I Hear? 41

2 Return to the Center: Balancing the Body
to Self-Regulate Orientation and Hearing   57
Human Consciousness and Hearing 59

Hearing Is a Learning Process   60
Locating the Source of Sound from a
   Reference Point   63
The Reference Point   65
The Body's Reactions to Stress   67
Let's Take a Look in the Mirror   68

3 Our Desire to Hear and Feel:
  Our Ears Connect Us to the World   77
  The World in Our Ears   80
  How Trauma Affects Hearing   84
  The 3 Types of Hearing Trauma   87
  It Hits Me: Where Do I Notice It in the Body?   93
  Disorders of the Ear   96

4 Everything Has a Beginning:
  The History of Sound Research   106
  All We Can Do We Once Learned   106
  What We Are Today Has Been Going on for
     Thousands of Years   108

5 The MUNDUS Method of Regenerating Hearing:
  The Step-by-Step Process   128
  Training Location to Rebuild Order   130
  EXERCISE: The Basic Therapeutic Method Using
     a Natural Sound Source   131
  The Basis for the Effects of the MUNDUS
     Basic Method   153
  Building Trust and Communication   158
  EXERCISE: The Basic Therapeutic Method Using
     a Natural Sound Transducer   158
  Conclusion to the Basic Method   180
  Part 1 Ends—Part 2 Begins   181

PART 2

The Journey Is the Goal
*Exercises that Further Support
Hearing Regeneration*

6 Being in the Present to Process the Past: Exercises
  to Find and Reflect On the Triggering Event   184
  The Three Central Pillars   184
  Tension and Balance   196
  If You Believe It, You Will See It!   199
  Resolving Trauma   200
  EXERCISE: Finding the Triggering Event   203

7 I Hear, Therefore I Am:
  Exercises to Recover Orientation   205
  Holograms Connect and Resonate with the World   206
  Regaining Vitality   208

8 Each Ship Has a Helmsman:
  Exercises to Take Control and Restore Order   210
  The Brain, Our Holographic Hub   211
  Our Body Stores All Our Experiences   212
  The Brain as Control Center   214
  Make Decisions That Work   216

9 No Pain, No Gain: Exercises for Resonance,
  Regulation, and Repetition   219
  Training Brings Knowledge to Action   219
  Everything Flows   221
  The Goal Is Integration   224
  Breaking Down Barriers   227
  Repetition of the Exercises   229

10 Nothing Is Impossible: One Step at a Time   234
    The Approach of Conventional Medicine and
      the Failure of Hearing Aids   240
    Training for Hearing Aid Users   245
    The Importance of Setting Goals   247
    In the Here and Now, Easily   250

11 A New Beginning: Four Principles for
   a Successful Life   252

APPENDIX A Directory of Exercises   256

APPENDIX B Reproducible Templates   258

            References   259

            About the Author   264

            Index   266

Acknowledgments

I WOULD LIKE TO SINCERELY THANK all those who have contributed to this book. My employees at MUNDUS GmbH helped me considerably: Frank Eberhardt, Mara Löffler, Katrin Löffler, and Mara Ebinger offered many hours of support throughout the process of preparing this book prior to publication. They read the text, discussed it with me, and helped me edit it. They put my sketches into printable form and were always willing to lend their knowledge and assistance.

The photographs of the exercises are intended to illustrate these processes as authentically as possible. For this I would like to thank our model, Milena Leonhardt, who displayed a naturalness that readily translates to the printed page.

Special thanks to my German publisher, AT Verlag, especially Urs Hunziker and Ralf Lay, who worked intensively with me to create the original edition of this book. As well, for facilitating a connection to AT Verlag, I have Dr. Anne Katharina Zschocke to thank. In an intensive conversation about my work she encouraged my impulse to put all my knowledge into a book. Thank you for your initiative and encouragement.

I am very grateful to my American publisher for its effort to bring my book into the English-speaking world. Special thanks from my heart go to Kayla Toher and Jeanie Levitan for their candor and patience to take into account all the subtle details of the concepts in this book and who cared for keeping the spirit of the English translation alive so that all people might apply the knowledge that is included in these pages.

Ines Helm has revised the manuscript with great sensitivity to make sure that the possibility of self-healing, based on the underlying laws of nature, has been translated into the English language, so every person, through understanding and training, is able to improve their sense of hearing.

My heartfelt thanks go to my partner, Jutta Ebinger, who is always right by my side with her big heart. She read the text with me for many months and helped me find the right words. Her feminine view of things enriches my life and has had an impact on this work in many ways.

Without all the people who have attended our seminars, getting involved in our work and strengthening it through their reports on their individual experiences, I would not have been able to penetrate so deeply and thoroughly into the heart of understanding inherent order. They have strengthened my confidence and have contributed to the deepening of my own knowledge and to the creation of this book. Thank you all!

Rebuilding Our Connection to the World

ONE MORNING AN ELDERLY WOMAN CALLED ME and asked, "I heard that you can improve your hearing, even at my age. Is that really true? And how does that work?"

In this book I will answer this question in a new way in the hope that it will remove any doubts or skepticism, such as "That can't be true; otherwise my doctor would have known about it," or "If I let my guard down and I'm disappointed again, that would be awful, because until now my experience has been that my hearing is getting worse, particularly in situations when it's noisy around me in a restaurant or when someone is talking next door. This has been going on for many years—and now you say my hearing can actually improve?"

Through hearing we have a special connection with everything that surrounds us—with the people we meet, with the birds that sing their songs, with the airplanes that fly above us, or with the pounding jackhammer on the road. We are in contact with all these things and many, many more through the sense of hearing.

Not being able to hear is not normal—not even when you get older. Yet it happens all too often, and as we shall soon learn it's usually as a result of stress or certain traumatic events in life. At some point we realize that we are constantly saying, "What did you say? Please say it again." Sometimes we add an apologetic "I'm sorry; it's so loud in here I can't understand you." Most likely you've not been satisfied with the answers you've received so far from the medical establishment. In searching for an alternative, you now hold this book in your hands, so at least you do hear your inner voice, and that's a good place to start.

This book is about how we can rebuild our sense of hearing naturally, step-by-step. Hearing doesn't regulate itself, so we need to understand the cause of hearing loss and adopt suitable training techniques that will restore this invaluable sense organ.

This book is the result of more than 10 years of practice during which I have worked closely with people who have all manner of hearing issues. I have drawn on the gifts and the experiences of my life, including my study of such diverse subjects as physics, biology, mathematics, medicine, and architecture. My teachers have been those who have looked deeply into their areas of expertise and have consistently explored our natural world, which we perceive and experience in our daily lives.

We are beings of flesh and blood; we each have a soul and spirit and follow life's physical laws. If we do not hear well, then we are, in a sense, in a state of imbalance. The aim of our work is to use the Basic Method of Hearing Regeneration to train our sense of hearing and add an impulse to further a sense of order within our **system** of body, spirit, and soul. In this case we'll be working with the **brain,** which initializes an order and the subsequent support for that directive. In this way we stimulate our **self-regulation,** which allows us to *find our center.*

System: A self-contained, ordered, and articulated whole; a totality, the structure or parts of which mesh, interact, and are interdependent (Greek, *Systema*)

Brain: The hub of the central nervous system in more sophisticated animals, especially vertebrates, in which the sensory centers and higher switching centers (coordination and association) are located. The brain is both an organ with a specific structure and complex functions that govern the physical control of our body, and a control center of our consciousness. It also has memory functions and possibilities of perception that we cannot specifically locate on an organic level.

Self-regulation: Control of oneself by oneself. The goal of most types of therapy is to improve an individual's ability to self-regulate; to gain (or regain) a sense of control over one's behavior and life.

An indispensable element in the basic method of hearing regeneration is a natural and well-defined sound source with which we can align ourselves. Such sounds can easily be found at home, for example, in the form of a running faucet, which is our preferred source. Through the method presented in this book, anyone can successfully train their hearing.

Sometimes such common sounds might not be enough to trigger our hearing, especially when there is significant hearing loss or other serious hearing issues, such as a one-sided hearing impairment or severe dizziness and increased sensitivity to noise (hyperacusis). Then it may be necessary to use a special speaker system in conjunction with the basic method taught in this book; namely, a natural sound transducer known in Europe as the Naturschallwandler (NSW), which I developed myself. This system emits sounds naturally as they occur in nature; that is, they radiate into three-dimensional space from a single point (for details refer to pages 37 through 41).

This book is aimed chiefly at those with mild onset hearing loss, although we will also look at more serious forms of hearing loss. I want to stress that even for those with serious conditions, the possibility of improvement always exists. A medical diagnosis that says you can't do anything about your hearing loss does not really mean the end of the road but rather can be the beginning of a whole new process for developing your supposedly impaired hearing.

We humans have an innate self-healing mechanism. Nature has given human beings the possibility of healing themselves, and this has been present long before any modern technology existed. For example, let's consider a middle-aged woman whom we worked with who had been diagnosed at age 4 with deafness in one ear. She underwent eight operations to improve her hearing—unfortunately, without any significant results. She resigned herself to the idea that there was nothing to be done, that her hearing was no longer functioning on an organic level. Yet we found that through the basic method outlined in this book she could once again develop a way for her deaf ear to perceive sounds. Of course, the basic method presented in this book does *not* lead to regrowth of the inner ear structure; however, it *does* help a person to more fully develop the capacity of their entire perceptual system so that you can "hear" even based on incomplete or only partially recognized information. As Johann Sebastian Bach so aptly said, "If we listen to music, the soul calculates."[1]

In this book I will show you how hearing works and how you can restore it naturally. The method is based on universal principles of physics. These principles describe forces that are noticeable and well described by science; for example, the law of gravity. You don't have to believe in gravity for it to operate in your life—you can simply observe its effects in your daily life. Thus, when working with principles of physics in the real world, you do not need to believe in them for them to be true. We can always trust this higher order of principles and are able to work with it since we are part of it. For a new way of seeing things, we have to be open to possibilities, for as Shakespeare's Hamlet says to his friend Horatio, "There are more things in heaven and earth than are dreamt of in your philosophy" (act 1, scene 5). This book is about real, concrete experiences. You don't have to believe what I say, because the proof is verifiable. It is not necessary to believe that gravity is there; you can easily check. Similarly, practicing the exercises in this book will be your proof as to whether the method works.

While the basic therapeutic method for hearing regeneration found in this book is based on certain principles of physics, which we are constantly connected to, there is another factor involved: our bodies have a higher-level mechanism by which we create conscious, controlled connections that help us function. This control mechanism is like a helmsman or captain. It can be described as our **awareness,** our *soul,* or our *divine quality.* Regardless of which term we use, this higher faculty allows us to develop our innate human potential for healing.

> **Awareness:** Mental clarity, consciousness, knowledge that something is happening or exists. Colloquially it refers to the state when we are awake or conscious. *Consciousness* is a complex concept, and its definition depends on the context in which it is used. For me, consciousness is knowledge from which follows ethical behavior. Awareness is the instance within us that perceives "I am." And the sum of all things of which I am aware, that I call *memory.* Our overall awareness also has another part that is understood as the *subconscious,* which is the aspect of the mind that is not obviously identified; for example, experiences that I've forgotten but that are still there.

THE THREE PILLARS OF THE METHOD

This method of self-healing is based on three central pillars:
- Body geometry
- Spatial localization
- Processing of perceptions

These are the three fundamental precepts on which we will focus. They are interconnected and depend on one another in a very precise and delicate manner to create our individual hearing profile. They form the basis of our physical reality and influence many processes of perception. When we reorient this control naturally, it brings about considerable self-regulatory effects by which we can develop our hearing capacity.

The results can be dramatic. People who have been told they need a hearing aid or who already wear one can return to using only their own ears to hear. In addition, there are other synergistic effects; for example, the case of 86-year-old Mr. Z, who now talks to his son at a normal volume. At the end of the training he said to me, "Well, Mr. Stucki, I have to tell you something! Since I started the training I often forget my cane because I feel much more confident on my feet!"

What I propose in this book is significantly linked to your hope for improvement in your ability to hear. Hope is critical, even if there has been one disappointment after another in search of solutions. And yet because you have this book in your hands, you must still have hope. It is vitally important to me that I explain the physical basis of our work as well as my experience with this method as accurately as possible. My intention is to make the explanations as clear as possible so that you can easily follow them by using your common sense. In this way you will understand why I claim that our faculty of hearing (and much else in our bodies) can rebuild itself. It is not about changing pathologies but instead about encouraging the basic ability to self-regulate. Yes, we can learn to hear again! We can learn to strengthen our innate self-healing powers, which is the goal of this book. The process is one of learning in stages, because as the Chinese proverb goes, "A journey of a thousand miles begins with a single step."

This book consists of 2 parts. In part 1, I explain the skills needed to create a foundation. In part 2, we build on this experience and knowledge.

When we learn new skills and apply them over and over again, we discover subtleties and aspects we did not notice the first time, when everything was new to us. Our perspective changes gradually as a result of repetition. The step-by-step ordering of chapters, the sections within chapters, and the exercises found throughout this book comprise a process that supports our system from different sides and systematically rebuilds our sense of hearing so as to regenerate its original qualities.

Incidentally, the previously mentioned elderly woman whom I

worked with has two hearing aids, which she now rarely uses. She now hears naturally and enjoys seminars, lectures, and training sessions because she hears and understands the presenters. She happily learns new things in life and loves passing this knowledge on to her friends and acquaintances. She is currently in training to help other people on their path in life.

I live and work in Germany. For the past 10 years, I have trained therapists in different European countries, mainly in German-speaking areas. I hope—with the help of translators—that I'll be able to train English-speaking therapists in the future as well. I'm prepared for and looking forward to teaching what I know all over the world, and I know there will be possibilities to achieve that.

Should you decide to undertake training in the method in a seminar setting, you'll have an opportunity to learn and practice the information presented here and clarify issues in a direct exchange with me. Dates and locations for trainings in central Europe are listed on the Naturschallwandler website, which can be translated into English using Google.

So, listen to your inner voice, the voice that told you to buy this book. Here you will find everything you need to retrain your hearing so that you can naturally hear and enjoy all the variety and beauty of sounds this world has to offer.

HOW TO USE THIS BOOK

I highly recommend that you use this book exactly as it is written, building your sense of hearing step-by-step as you gradually add to your knowledge. Practice the exercises where they are described before going on to the next section or the next exercise. In other words, don't skip through the instructions.

This book is aimed at all people and can be used for yourself or for the support of others to help them improve their sense of hearing.

A Note on "I," "You," and "We"

You will notice that I change pronouns throughout this book. Sometimes I write from the perspective of "I," then I might say "you," and I also speak of "we."

- When I use the pronoun "I," I am referring to each individual reader in his or her own realm of experience from an individual perspective. I do this because I want to encourage the reader to internalize what has been written and realize that it applies to them personally. It is not a hint that only applies to others. (Sometimes "I" also refers to me as the author.)
- When I use "you," I mean you, the reader, or you, the person for whom the work is intended from the view of the therapist or the training partner.
- "We" is always a reference to the interaction between "me" and "you." It reflects our common interaction and cooperation as well as the mutual effects that result. "We" is also all of us in unity on our home planet. No one person or point of view is better than another—we are just in different places and have different points of view. And we can, if we want to, change these positions and move

into new ones. When I speak of "we," I mean it inclusively. I use this term when I am speaking of the generally accepted rules and structures that apply to all of us. Pain is individually perceived; the mechanism of healing, however, is universally similar for everyone. But everything always depends on our individual attitude, our intentions, our focus, and ultimately our decisions.

A Note on Participant Examples

I thought long and hard about which real-life experiences with participants I wanted to share in this book. Some of the stories shared about working with the exercises and our Naturschallwandler may sound too good to be true. Of course, you want to know: Does it work? Therefore, examples are helpful proof. However, they are often associated with some pressure, because in the beginning of the work you are not yet at the end results of those stories. And if I tell you now that we can always achieve an improvement, you might think, "It sounds too good to be true." But I assure you it is a fact. When we begin to lift weights or go walking daily, our body becomes stronger. I do not have to believe in this, for it is just basic physics. Our hearing can become stronger too. It has nothing to do with belief; it is pure physics.

For both the person who experiences an improvement, as well as for the person accompanying the participant, the experiences gained through the work with these exercises are gifts. Sometimes changes are very fast—sometimes they take time to occur. Everyone is different, so your own experience will be different. It is not about taking the examples as benchmarks to achieve something specific, and it's not about having to reach for something in particular. The examples are meant to motivate you on your own path toward achieving your own improvements and developments.

Numbers Are Numbers

In this book I have written quantities as Arabic numerals rather than spelling them out. Numbers have a symbolism all their own. Each figure

· ٩ ۲۲ ٤ ٥۲ ۷٨٩

· ١ ۲ ۳ ٤ ٥٦ ۷٨٩

In Europe, 2 was rotated by 180 degrees and 3 was rotated by 90 degrees to bring about their present form:

0   1   2   3   4   5   6   7   8   9

is a signal that acts on us with its unique symbolism. The 10 digits with which we write all numbers are of Indian origin[2] and have been handed down to us as symbol characters taken from the Arabic culture.

The first 4 figures after 0 (1, 2, 3, 4) add up to the number 10. The number 10 expresses a new level. The numbers 0–9 can be written in one stroke, but the number 10 has to be written in 2 steps because it's made of 2 numbers. The numbers 0 to 9 follow an inner logic. There is a sense in their order, and they explain something about creation and how things manifest in our world. The number 10 is an abstraction of this original order and therefore reveals a new plane. This is the base 10 or decimal system.

The numeral forms are processed in our perception and in our consciousness differently than the spelled-out numbers one, two, three, four. The Old Testament, in the original Jewish tradition known as the Torah, was handed down from generation to generation and is written using 22 Hebrew letters, each of which represents a specific numerical value with associated meanings.[3] Numbers are something universal and tell a story. This meaning changes when I write a number as a word.

Numbers written as numbers show clearly defined relationships of space and surface. Many of us remember the Pythagorean theorem $a^2 + b^2 = c^2$. This formula can be written with numbers as small as 3, 4, and 5: $3^2 + 4^2 = 5^2$. With these figures, ancient builders constructed their right angles in temples and buildings. The correlation between numbers and space can also be found in the process of regenerating our sense of hearing.

The Basics and the Basic Method

Understanding Hearing Loss and the Potential for Regeneration

1

A Great Start Means Knowing Where You're Going

Orientation to the Basics

ALL BIOLOGICAL BEINGS HAVE THE ABILITY to heal themselves. This includes human beings. We all have experienced this day after day from the time we were babies. We stub our toe on the table leg, cut our finger, or knock our ankle against the wall. It hurts, maybe it bleeds, but it immediately compels our body to start a healing process. After an injury, the body immediately starts its inherent **regulation** and **regeneration** process. This capability is part of all living things. A machine is not able to do the same. Sometimes, however, we notice that this natural healing process is either very slow or not moving along, or the healing is not complete. It's then that we realize that our body is not working as efficiently as it did before the injury.

> **Regulation, regulate:** control; organize; make even; according to a standard, a measure; a level set (Latin, *regula,* "scale"). I use this term to refer to the automatic adaptation of a living being to a natural state of order, which is homeostasis, the tendency of the elements or groups of elements of an organism to come into equilibrium. Regulation is a process. Where there is a physical dysfunction or injury, the stabilization of symptoms to achieve a

balance is the primary goal in the beginning; from there, further healing can take place.

Regeneration: Recovery, renewal, the natural replacement of lost organic parts. Regeneration is a way to restore any living organism, including the organic parts and functions of the body. It is our inherent healing capability: the body can heal itself.

In this book we consider the regulation and regeneration process as it pertains specifically to hearing: Why do we hear worse? Why do we no longer hear as we did before? What are the causes of hearing loss? How can we regulate and regenerate our whole, unified system—our body with all its features, as well as our soul or spirit and our mind? How can we strengthen and activate our capabilities to restore skills that have been lost, or gain new ones? A healthy system responds and always works as an integrated whole. If parts are adversely affected, this will impact the whole system.

Although complete healing must also take place on a spiritual level, it is not absolutely necessary for someone to have a strong connection to the spiritual dimension of healing for this method to work. In the final analysis it is the actual physical experience of healing that is the proof of the effectiveness of this method. Knowledge of the method and awareness of the intention behind it are all that are needed to rebuild the structures for hearing that will allow the healing powers within to flow so that we can hear ourselves and the voices around us once more. The capacity for self-healing is a basic human capability, and it is simply on this that we are building. It applies to hearing as well as all other functions of the body.

In this book I draw on the theoretical basis for the regeneration of hearing. I explain the **basic method** that has been in practical use since 2009. The theory and procedures are complemented by practical exercises that can be easily implemented at home, either alone or with the assistance of a partner. The practical approach presented in this book is novel, unconventional, and connects different areas of knowledge in the fields of physiology, biology, anatomy, physics, psychology, trauma therapy, **field theory,** and brain research. This approach goes beyond the purely mechanical notion that damage to the mechanism in the ear and subsequent hearing loss are the result of bent hairs in the inner ear or other such theories. It is truly possible to improve one's hearing, no matter what.

> **Basic method:** This is the proprietary method of training in consecutive steps to bring about improvement in listening skills. The term MUNDUS Basic Method for Listening Regeneration is trademarked in Germany at the German Patent and Trademark Office.

> **Field theory:** A model describing physical reality by means of fields, examining the interaction between the individual and the total field, or environment. Field theory applies to both psychology and physics. Classical field theory works especially with mathematics to describe the physical forces and their interactions. Rupert Sheldrake, former research fellow of the Royal Society and former director of studies in biochemistry and cell biology at Clare College, Cambridge University, developed the concept of morphogenetic (formative) fields, which describe survival-related information of living beings in nonmaterial so-called information fields. These are available to all beings, especially those of the same species.[1]

I ask you to consider whether this approach has a real impact, if it ultimately improves your hearing and your world. If you get to a point where you stop working on improving your hearing through this method because you're having trouble understanding the method, you are welcome to contact me with any questions you may have. In the end it's all about listening to one another. And if you only find inspiration in this book, this too is wonderful!

EACH PERSON CAN HEAR

Blindness cuts us off from things, but deafness cuts us off from people . . .

HELEN KELLER

We are not hard of hearing—we just do not hear where the other person is.

Are you familiar with this situation? You speak to someone alone in a quiet room. They talk in a normal voice, maybe even quietly, and you can understand each other perfectly. However, it is quite different when you're talking with someone and it is a bit noisy around you; for example, in a crowded restaurant. Everyone is talking and music blares from speakers on the ceiling and the walls. Now you have a problem: you can barely follow the conversation at your own table.

Or let's say you're sitting at a large table, perhaps on a conference call that's attended by several people. The conversation goes back and forth, and it is of course particularly important to hear who is speaking. To hear who is speaking you must concentrate and may miss your turn to have a say. Before you realize what was said, the next person has already begun to speak, and you have lost the thread of the conversation, as well your connection to the others.

Conclusion: On a one-to-one basis I can hear and understand the other person, but if other noise sources are added I do not clearly understand what's being said. This tells us two things:

- Basically, we can hear, because otherwise we would not be able to understand the other person in a one-on-one interaction.
- We find it difficult to focus on a single source when we have multiple sources of noise occurring at the same time. Why this is and how we can learn to hear others better even when there are multiple sources of noise will be explained in the following chapters.

By listening, we want to understand—what are we hearing? We listen to one another, and we listen to ourselves. We want to understand in ourselves what the world "out there" is telling us. This is a very complex process, by which many **aspects** of our senses interact and work together.

> **Aspect:** Sight, viewpoint, perspective; essential elements of a particular status or phase from which something is regarded; for example, from an individual's specific emotions, physical condition, or acquired skills (Latin, *aspectus*, "the inspection" or "the look")

The structure of the ear that enables the hearing process is summarized as follows:

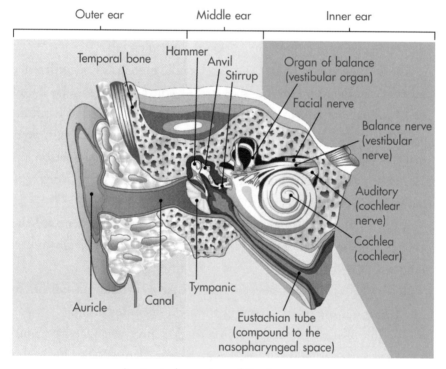

Anatomical overview of the human ear

Information in the form of sound waves and vibrations coming from an outside source meet our anatomical organ of hearing. The ears act as a shell that receives sound waves and directs them inward, to the ear canal.

There, the sound waves strike the eardrum, causing it to vibrate. Connected directly to the eardrum are the three smallest and hardest bones found in this structure: the hammer, the anvil, and the stirrup. These structures pass the movement through the inner tubes to the cochlea. Here, waves are triggered by changes in pressure, which in turn set the hair cells in motion, like wind moving the tops of the trees in the forest.

Each one of these approximately 20,000 to 30,000 hair cells (the figures vary greatly) in the **cochlea** (part of the inner ear) is connected to a nerve cell, and these nerve cells pass the stimulation obtained as an electrical pulse via the auditory nerve to the brain. The first stop is the brain stem, so as to respond quickly if necessary. From there the stimulation goes into different areas of the brain.[2]

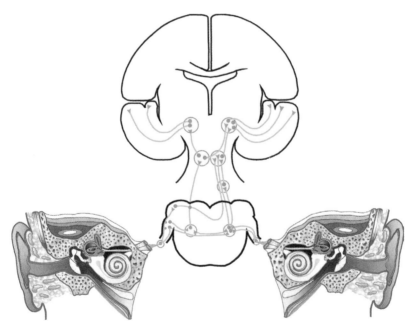

The path of sound (i.e., information) traveling from the ear to the brain, a complex path of signal transduction. The circles with dots represent clusters of nerve cells, in effect a "data center" where information in the form of sound is first evaluated and processed. The yellow lines represent the nerve fibers, which are more numerous on the right side. This entire route is the "hearing superhighway." We know a lot about the anatomy of hearing, but we don't yet know how it all plays together and how it's possible that this multitude of nerves and nerve conduction structures matches up with one another and still processes information in a fraction of second.

> **Cochlea:** Part of the inner ear (Greek, *kochlias,* meaning "screw, screw-shaped structure")

Also involved in hearing is our vestibular system (the semicircular canals in the figure above that are responsible for balance), which sits in the ear and gives the finest control pulses via the balance nerve into our muscles.

Each ear is connected to both halves of the brain—technically, cross-connected—and affects the basic electrical vibration of our brain, which can be seen in an **EEG.** The hearing process thus influences how the two halves of the brain interact and work together optimally.

> **EEG:** Abbreviation for *electroencephalogram* or *electroencephalography* (Greek, *egkephalon,* "brain"). EEGs are noninvasive and record the electrical activity of the brain.

We also hear low frequencies through our bones (called *bone conduction*). On the other hand, high vibrations, in particular air-pressure fluctuations, are perceived by our body tissues, especially the skin. Even deaf people who do not or no longer consciously perceive spoken sounds feel their vibrations and process them. All living beings, from the smallest microbe to the largest whale, can hear; that is, they perceive vibrations, process them, react to them, and even give their own specific vibration in response in the form of words, singing, bubbling, barking, or other sound responses.

For humans, hearing is inseparable from speech, with the perception of our environment and our information—our vibration—our message to the world. When I hear the joyful laughter of my child, I relax. When I hear the pervasive *nee-naw* of fire engines, my attention and my tension immediately increase. In the first situation, my heartbeat slows down and my blood pressure drops; in the second, my heart beats faster and my blood pressure rises to be able to react if necessary. Thus sounds provide a constantly changing landscape. They influence our lives and determine how we feel, whether we relax or go on alert. Our whole system of perception is involved. My hearing is constantly in the "on" mode. Even when I sleep, I react to noises. We don't ever stop listening. As soon there is an unusual sound, our bodies awaken. Our consciousness constantly scans the environment through the sense of hearing, processing the information both near and far to determine whether everything is alright. That's precisely why our hearing is also responsible for our body's sense of security: because through hearing we perceive things that we do not see.

Our hearing is 360 degrees, so it's an all-around sense, going in all directions. We can look through a window when we're in a room; however, this is only a limited perception of our environment. But we can even hear through walls. We know what goes on around us. I can hear people talking in the other room, even when the TV is on or someone is yelling, "Where are you?" outside the door, even though I do not see the source of the sound.

How quickly we switch from relaxation to maximum alertness can be seen in many old Western films: As the good guys sit around the campfire in the evening, quietly talking and eating, the bad guys sneak up to ambush them. As a branch cracks upon their approach, all the good guys suddenly jump up and go on alert. Sensing danger, their hearing is acute. A less dramatic example is our reaction to an alarm clock, set at a certain pitch so that our perceptual system is alerted when it goes off, taking us from sleep to wakefulness.

THE PROCESS OF HEARING

Note: This section includes some technically detailed information aimed generally at professionals and laypeople with a strong interest in this kind of detail. Please bear in mind that this level of technical information is not required for a basic understanding of the method taught in this book.

A healthy sense of hearing facilitates (via acoustic perception) your correct and complete **orientation** in a **room.** Your spatial awareness in relation to other static or moving bodies within the whole spectrum of your surroundings is determined via your sense of hearing, which is calculated instantly in the brain. This defines your physical position, your own point of view in three-dimensional space and time. The temporal sequence—which noise follows another, how long an object needs to reach me or move past me—is important information that you receive via the sense of hearing.

> **Orientation:** The act or process of determining a direction or determining one's location (French, *orienter*, "contact"); with regard to the hearing, the exact position of a noise source in space

> **Room:** Dimension; length, width, and height; space, possibly something that accommodates; real space such as a bedroom or living room; mental space

The movements of ourselves and others, as well as the speed of motion or motionlessness, are recorded via the sense of hearing, then transmitted through the central nervous system to the auditory center in the brain, where it is evaluated and calculated. We have seen that each inner ear is connected to both sides of the brain. Thus, for example, acoustic signals coming from both ears are compared with each other in the brain. The differences between the same signal in the left and right ears are analyzed, and from this our brain calculates the movement of the source of the sound. At the same time, the content of the sound is evaluated: Is it, for example, a fire engine?

Location, orientation, and sequence are closely linked. The acoustic location takes place via a three-dimensional axis system, which differentiates between:

Front and back = horizontal axis
Top and bottom = vertical axis
Right and left = lateral axis

So that the brain can calculate the position and motion of an object properly, it needs precise, physically correct, acoustically unique information about what's being heard. If the hearing is impaired or it provides confusing information to the brain, the correct and clear calculation of acoustic information in the environment is compromised, and the clear orientation and processing of the information is thus impeded. This is what we call bad or compromised hearing. Auditory information is hindered. We subjectively experience this as "poor listening."

But it's not normal for one's hearing to get worse, not even when you get older. Yet, as we know, for many people it is a reality. And it's not only our ability to perceive very fine or very quiet sounds that we lose, such as the buzzing of a fly in a room or the sound of leaves gently rustling in the wind. As much as we may miss those subtler sounds of life, this level of hearing sensitivity is not critical to our main human-to-human communication, which is comparatively louder.

This is all to say that measuring sound is quite complicated, and the values are not as objective as we might wish. An acoustic master once told me, "With all our programs, with their curves and measured values, we determine whether people are able to hear well or not. Everything else mainly is so changeable that we often get very different values from one measurement to the next."

The table on the next page presents an overview of various noises and their volume as measured in **decibels** (dB) that our sense of hearing perceives within a certain spectrum. This unit was named *bel* in honor of scientist and inventor Alexander Graham Bell (1847–1922), who is famous for advancing ideas that brought the telephone to market. This measurement unit is not about absolute values but rather about the ratio of two measured values to each other; for example, a TV on low volume (60 dB) compared with the noise of heavy traffic (70 dB). Of course, the distance from the noise source is always the crucial factor. Therefore, always consider measured values as a function of proximity to the source. This scale of values is a **logarithmic function.** This means that every 10 dB value is doubled. A value of 40 dB is thus not 4 times louder than the initial value of 10 dB but rather 8 times louder.

EXAMPLES OF SOUNDS AND THEIR VOLUME IN DB (DECIBELS)[3]

	Value	Unit of measure	All 10 dB volume doubled	Factor of the increase from baseline in:	
				Good	Weakened hearing (−30 dB)
Just audible sound	10	dB(A)*	10	x 1	
Soft rustle of leaves	15–20	dB(A)	20	x 2	
Whisper, one's own breathing sound	30	dB(A)	30	x 4	x 1
Quiet residential area	30–40	dB(A)	40	x 8	x 2
Quiet conversation, quiet office	40–50	dB(A)	50	x 16	x 4
Normal conversation Speech level, the area of greatest information content to the human ear	50–60	dB(A)	60	x 32	x 8
TV on low volume	60	dB(A)			
Heavy traffic	70–80	dB(A)	70	x 64	
Shouting	80–85	dB(A)	80	x 128	
Van passing by; lawnmower distance of 10 m	85–90	dB(A)	90	x 256	
Jackhammer distance of 10 m; music through headphones	90–100	dB(A)	100	x 512	
Nightclub (average value)	92–111	dB(A)		x 1,024	
Express train passing by; printing house (i.e., for newspapers)	100–110	dB(A)	110		
Steel forge	110–120	dB(A)	120		
Propeller plane at distance of 3 m	120–130	dB(A)	130		
Shot	132–173	dB(A)			
Jet at distance of 30 m	150	dB(A)	140		

*The label (A) denotes the frequency value of the sound pressure level decibel. The level of loudness our brain perceives depends on the frequencies contained in the sound, and our brain is less sensitive to very low or very high frequency sounds. The label (A) shows at what decibel our brain perceives the sound to be. This measurement is a type of "weighting filter" that measures sound more like the human ear. The frequency value is a deduction or surcharge-determined level and is the "weighted sound pressure level," called dB(X) or dBx. The symbol X stands for the specifically set weighted filter used in each case. Weighting filters common in practical applications are the A-weighting, expressed as dB(A), and at high sound pressure levels the C rating, or dB(C).

Decibel: A unit for expressing the ratio of two amounts of electric or acoustic signal power equal to 10 times the common logarithm of this ratio (Latin, *decem*, "ten"); a unit for expressing the relative intensity of sounds on a scale from 0 for the average least-perceptible sound, to about 130 for the average pain level; a degree of loudness

Logarithmic function, logarithm: The number with which one multiplies the number a in the equation $a^b = c$ to obtain the number c (Greek, *logos*, "reason ratio," and *arithmos*, "number"); the exponent that indicates the power to which a base number is raised to produce a given number, e.g., the logarithm of 100 to the base 10 is 2

Clue to the Connection between How People Experience Noise and Which Results Will Be Measured Technically When Noise Is Produced[4]

+10 dB is the level of the doubly perceived loudness in psychoacoustics, which describes the human sensations in sound events and their relationship to actual measured values—in other words, how humans perceive sounds and the psychological and physiological responses associated with them. The lower the volume, the finer we perceive the differences.

+6 dB corresponds to a doubling in the sound pressure (voltage) at the measured level change of +6 dB.

+3 dB level increase requires twice the energy; that is, the amplifier power calculated predominantly.

Any noise will be heard twice as loud when it is just +10 dB louder than before. When the noise was produced technically (for example, by an amplifier), the pressure of noise doubles when it's just +6 dB louder than before, and the energy needed doubles when the sound has risen +3 dB. This shows that there is a substantial difference between how nature produces sound and how established equipment produces sound.

The table on page 22 shows that despite a weakening of hearing (auditory threshold at 30 dB), we should still hear a conversation conducted at a normal volume, as this is still 8 times louder than the sound of normal breathing. That means that even with already advanced hearing loss, if we only have a hearing perception above 40 dB, a conversation would still be 4 times louder than the sounds that we can normally hear.

Once again, what I would like to make clear is this: If I do not understand my interlocutor because I did not hear her correctly—that is, if even a normal-volume conversation for my sense of hearing is not loud enough—it very rarely involves what we think of as deafness. And yet it happens often that I may experience "difficult listening." That's because we "unlearn" how to hear properly because of certain events in life, specifically, traumatic events (a subject we'll explore in more detail later).

Our task, therefore, is to learn how to hear again. We can rebuild our sense of hearing by training the brain in acoustic detection and processing of auditory information. For this we don't need to regrow or replace anything. The hardware—the physical components that comprise our sense of hearing—is already in the state it is in. Our task is to relearn how to fully and correctly use this hardware. How and why this works to restore hearing is explained in stages in this book, and the precise instructions for training (the MUNDUS Basic Method for Listening Regeneration) are found in chapter 5, while strengthening exercises are described in chapters 6 through 10.

THE ABILITY TO LEARN THROUGH TRAINING

The perception of our individual world, both the world "out there" and our internal world, is shaped by our consciousness. This is the aspect of our being that perceives, compares, and differentiates. It's our method of using knowledge that we've already acquired or are in the process of acquiring. The processing of information that we already know is automatic and requires very little of our attention; for example, shifting gears while driving or riding a bicycle. Once we have learned such skills and repeated them often enough, we can do them casually without thinking about them. So in general we are well equipped for the learning process. Even young people have physiological structures that have evolved over millions of years in the course of human evolution. This ability to learn is wonderfully suited to adapting to change and is self-regulating.

However, in the course of learning something new, information that puts too great of a strain on us is often excluded either in whole or in part. For example, when we are learning how to read as small children, we're under a certain amount of pressure to learn, and we might even have been subjected to criticism for not learning fast enough ("I don't know why you're so slow!"). This kind of pressure can be too much for the current life stage in which we find ourselves, so the new information is placed in the subconscious, where it is not directly accessible.

Each function and skill we can control today we could not control right off the bat. Let's look at a child who is taking her first steps. How many steps have to be mastered, how often does she fall down and get up, over and over again, until she has learned fine motor control, orientation, and the control of individual muscle groups? The same is true with hearing. As a rule, we are born with a very fine ear attuned to the world, but we must first learn how to process sounds and assign meaning to them. Children do this automatically. How? Among other ways, through one of their favorite games, hide-and-seek. This, incidentally, is a very good exercise for adults as well.*

---

*A list of all exercises that facilitate our relearning hearing can be found in appendix A.

(((•))) EXERCISE: Playing Hide-and-Seek

This exercise is fun and can be played indoors or outdoors, in any weather. It's the familiar childhood game of hide-and-seek: "Where are you? I hear you . . . I'm coming." So you playfully learn to locate sounds in space.

If we have lost an ability or we have not learned it yet, regardless of what kind of ability, we can relearn it step-by-step. We can train. In relearning a skill it's important to follow proper procedure so you can regain the desired capability in successive, consecutive steps. This is true of hearing. Training is the main way we work on regenerating our sense of hearing. You may say, "I'm always listening—am I always in training?" No. If we no longer hear well, we're not in training; we're burdened. For example, say I've strained my back and that has resulted in pain. It hurts, so I avoid using that part of my body, and consequently I adopt a more protective posture, which may cause a distorted pose. Nevertheless I say to myself, *I still have to do something to train, go running, jogging, whatever.* If I move from resolution to action, then in reality I've created a physical stress because my body cannot implement the action. Only when my back has healed again does it makes sense to go for a walk or a jog. Then it does my body good and strengthens it.

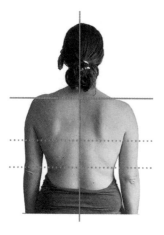

*Example of the consequences of a change in posture. Vertical axis: The head is shifted to the right. The right shoulder hangs, therefore the upper body is displaced and is in tension (shoulder blades and arms are not at the same height). This 34-year-old mother of three children often has back pain and tension, which has resulted in bilateral **tinnitus** and hearing loss.*

Tinnitus: The general term for subjectively perceived noise in the ears such as bells, murmurs, and whistles (Latin, *tinnitus*, "ringing, clicking")

It is the same with hearing. If I am not centered (the connection is explained at the end of this chapter), then the area where my auditory sensation occurs is not well oriented or balanced, and hearing is a burden. Hearing is exhausting for me and prolonged listening tires me—even when what I hear interests me. Therefore, our task is to rebuild a natural order; that is, to bring a healthy impulse into an existing imbalance with the aim of restoring our natural sense of perception.

RELEARNING THE HEARING PROCESS

Our ability to perceive is connected to a central control that coordinates all processes of perception as well as the processing and execution of bodily functions. This central control is our conscious being. On the physical level, this awareness is represented by the many individual cells of the brain and the nervous system combined. Body awareness works even when we sleep. The physical aspect of our total consciousness operates largely autonomously and instinctively, with information anchored in our genes, ensuring the survival of our organism. Our consciousness also consists of another aspect, which has been described as the "soul," the "spirit," and the "mind" (as distinct from the brain). This aspect is not bound by the body and can experience things independent of the body; for example, when we imagine or visualize something in great detail.

Both aspects of consciousness are always in exchange with each other, learning from each other. In doing so, our mind works like a computer program to automate processes and the processing of information (such as walking). Notably, these programs can be rewritten by our consciousness (relearned); we can change an existing skill or delete a skill that's no longer needed or long forgotten.

To improve our consciousness as a control entity and thus strengthen the basis for relearning how to hear, we follow three central pillars, which will be explored in detail in subsequent chapters:

- **Body geometry:** This defines the balance and symmetry of our body along the vertical and horizontal axes. Our body geometry stores and reflects all our experiences and traumas.
- **Spatial localization:** How do we find our way in the world? Where is everything? Can we orient ourselves, or are we confused because things are not where we expect them to be? Do we perceive sounds from where they originate, or are we always surprised? "Oh, that's where it comes from—I thought I heard it from somewhere else."
- **Processing of perception:** What does our brain do with the information it receives? Why does processing sometimes seem not to work so well?

These three pillars are directly involved in all processes of hearing. They influence and support one another in a very precise and subtle way. If one of them doesn't work optimally, then our hearing is weakened. They affect many other processes of perception as well as the physical functioning of the body.

If our control mechanism, our consciousness, is realigned on the basis of these three pillars, we can achieve considerable self-regulation. The basic therapeutic method I have developed, described in detail in chapter 5, involves these three pillars. Improvements in hearing impairment of all kinds can be achieved because this method is based on physical principles that apply to all people. But first let's look at the fascinating physical fundamentals of sound.

Experiencing Balance

As mentioned in the introduction, an 86-year-old gentleman of the "old school" said to me after three training sessions, "So, Mr. Stucki, let me tell you something! Ever since I've started training, I often forget my cane because I feel much more confident on my feet!" He smiled at me.

His son, a therapist in the resolution of trauma, added, "My father

can move much better and no longer has too many balance problems."
Besides that, they could better connect with one another again. If he
had not witnessed this himself, he would never believe it.

PHYSICS AND ACOUSTICS

We cannot go wrong if we follow nature.

MICHEL DE MONTAIGNE

Natural acoustics is the physical process that results in the formation
and propagation of sounds as they occur naturally, without any manipulation by humans or by human technology. The teacher of natural
acoustics is Nature herself.

The word *acoustic* originates from the Greek word *akoustikos,* "of
or for hearing, ready to hear." Acoustics is the branch of physics that
deals with the study of sound. It is concerned with all phenomena that
are perceptible to the ear, with the connections between the formation
and generation of sound, with its propagation, and with its influence
and analysis. Other components of acoustic theory are the interaction
of sound with certain materials and the perception of sound through
hearing, including its effects on humans and animals. Acoustics is an
interdisciplinary field that is closely linked to other disciplines, including physics, psychology, physiology, and **materials science.**

> **Materials science:** Also called *materials science and engineering,*
> this is an interdisciplinary field that deals with the structural
> arrangement of materials and substances and their mechanical,
> physical, and chemical properties.

Let us now turn to the fundamental laws of acoustics. Naturally produced sounds and noises, including the sounds of musical instruments
and the human voice, physically spread in spherical sound fields. Starting
from one point, all frequencies of the sound image move simultaneously

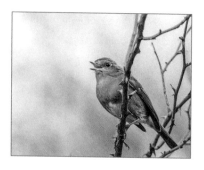

A bird sings a song, and our heart connects to it. Photo by Paul Heidemann.

in all directions in space. A sound in nature—the gentle splashing of a creek, the song of a bird in the forest, or the playing of a violin—can be heard clearly and precisely throughout the environment.

A bird in the forest sings a song, and something else happens: the stomata of nearby plants open and the gas exchange is enhanced, which affects the growth and health of the plants.[5] Meanwhile, we can hear the bird equally well from almost all directions. The direct sound component—the sound emitted through the bird's mouth or beak, almost in one direction—only makes up a small percentage of the total sound component of the bird's song, about 10 to 15 percent. The shape of the sound-generating body dictates whether the direct sound component increases (like a trumpet) or diminishes (like a singing bowl or violin) based on the design. The trumpet sends the sound into the world whereas the singing bowl or violin keeps the sound contained.

Should I move farther away from the bird, its song, though now quieter to my ears, still remains intact, as it was before. Technically, hardly any of the bird's frequencies are lost, hence there is a natural propagation principle at work. A conventional sound-system speaker, however, does not work the same way as the bird. The farther away from the speaker I move, the more its frequencies are lost, even if I am still orientated toward the speaker. For example, we don't hear clear sound from an open-air concert if we're at a distance, only a more or less diffused booming sound, especially coming from the bass, which emits lower frequencies. The little bird sings with only a few watts, yet its frequencies are more far-reaching. A conventional speaker works with a lot more energy than a bird does, yet it doesn't have the same far-reaching effect. This phenomenon has nothing to do with the quality of the speaker either.

The principle of propagation in all directions is fundamental. We experience an omnipresence in the spreading of sounds waves—no direction is preferred. Gravity works like that too, and beams of light shine in all directions. It's much like light waves, wherein each atom of light has a kind of center that gathers electrons in a defined order that radiates in all directions.

Sound is a force of nature and is in many aspects subject to the four fundamental interactions, or fundamental forces of nature, the interactions that do not appear to be reducible to more basic interactions. These are:

- weak interaction,
- strong interaction,
- electromagnetic interaction, and
- gravitational interaction.

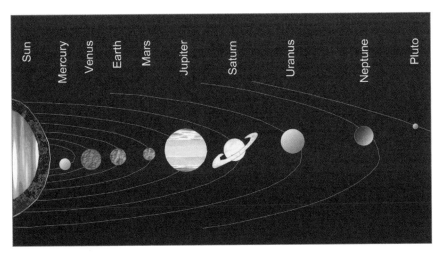

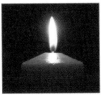 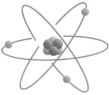

Examples from nature of the propagation of energy and order from a single point: planetary system, candle (light), atom (model)

Although it is possible to describe these forces, they still cannot be explained and completely understood. Similarly,

> When we pluck a note on the string of a violin, the string begins to vibrate and the note is carried by the air to our ears. This is a curious phenomenon. The gas molecules collide with each other in the same way as billiard balls. The number of molecules in a liter of gas is unimaginably high (approximately 10^{22}). When an entire orchestra plays in a hall, the confusion that reigns in the molecules of the air is so enormous that every explanation to date for explaining sound transmission is inadequate. The music that reaches us from the stage and is reflected a thousand-fold on walls, ceiling, rows of seats, etc., should really hit our ears as an unbearable screeching. Instead infinitely precise information reaches our eardrums, whether as vibrations or through the medium of electrical signals.[6]

Now imagine that no matter where you are in a room with the singing bird (above, below, to the side), its song, a source of information, is transmitted in all directions. Viewed as a form of energy, this means that this force, this song, is distributed throughout the room, similar to the way the sun's energy radiates light in all directions. The farther we are from the source, an ever-decreasing amount of energy remains. Nevertheless, we still hear the bird's frequencies clearly over long distances.

Let's consider the example of throwing two stones side by side into water. We see how each wave freely unfolds, with the waves penetrating one another instead of displacing one another, such that each stone's waves move within the circles of the other stone's waves. This applies even if the stones are thrown with varying force, one after the other, into the water, resulting in different wave crests.

When I throw a stone in the water, concentric waves form, spreading out in ripples on the water's surface. The same principle applies to sound. Since sound waves always propagate spatially, their waves are always three-dimensional. So two (or more) different sounds, like two

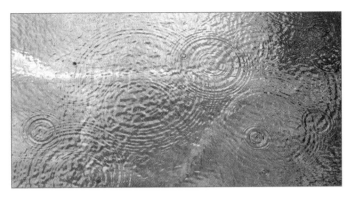

Mutually penetrating water circuits

different stones thrown in the water, will, in a sense, overlap in concentric waveforms. This is called a *spherical sound wave.*

This brings us to an important principle: *natural waves penetrate one another without erasing or displacing anything.* In nature, one event is never completely identical to another. They can be very similar, but they're never exactly the same. Any natural wave traveling at the same time as other waves in the same space will be different in terms of their strength, including their **amplitude** (wave height), **frequency** (the distance from wave peak to wave peak), and their propagation speed in space. A single frequency can be deleted, but not the wave itself, which consists of different individual frequencies. Here we recognize the principle of *zero pressure,* wherein sound waves propagate almost without pressure and evenly in three-dimensional space, overlapping harmoniously and flowing into one another without displacing one another.

Amplitude: The extent of a vibratory movement measured from the mean position to an extreme; the maximum departure of a value of an alternating wave from the average value (Latin, *amplus,* "ample")

Frequency: The number of complete oscillations per second of energy (such as sound or electromagnetic energy) in the form of waves (Latin, *frequentia,* "numerous")

These facts about sound waves are valid for all kinds of natural waves. Sound waves can have a wide variety of frequencies, from very low, just over the range of audible (infrasonic), to the human hearing range (from 15 all the way up to 20,000 hertz), to extremely high frequencies (ultrasound). Humans can perceive frequencies that are outside the range audible by the ear, meaning that sound is not only perceived by the ear but also by the bones and even through the skin. In fact, humans are able to perceive frequencies with their whole organism, even the frequencies outside their hearing range.

Another fundamental quality of natural sound is its ability to penetrate matter, to flow through it and leave an effect. Expressions such as "His voice cuts right through me" or "The music touches my heart" describe sensations that are not just **metaphorically** understood but that also reflect an actual physiological fact.

Metaphor: A figure of speech rather than literally denoting an idea or object (Greek, *metapherein*, "to transfer")

To summarize, three principles of natural sound propagation are:
- sound radiates from one point and travels outward in all directions,
- sound propagates free of pressure, and
- sound penetrates matter.

Another aspect of natural sound induction is the separation of the excitation point and the radiator. The example of a violin illustrates this point.

There is always a point at which a sound is produced, which is the excitation point, and a surface or body that radiates the generated sound into the environment, which is the radiator. The excitation point is spatially separated from the radiating body, as in the case of the violin. The strings of the violin are vibrated with the stroke of a bow and produce a **sound** wave. This sound wave, when generated only by the strings, is relatively quiet, just as it would be on a harp, which radiates sound directly from the strings.

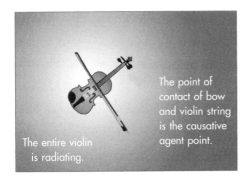

The point of contact of bow and violin string is the causative agent point.

The entire violin is radiating.

The point of contact of a bow scraping the violin string is the causative agent, or excitation point. The entire violin body is the radiator, sending sound out in waves.

Sound: A particular auditory impression; the sensation perceived by the sense of hearing; in musical instruments, the vibrations of amplifying bodies (Latin, *sonus,* "sound")

The point at which the stroke of a bow touches the violin strings is the excitation point of the sound. Once the string is vibrated, the sound waves pass through the body of the violin, which radiates the sound. In this process, certain frequencies in the **resonance** body of the instrument are erased or amplified as determined by the shape of the violin body (the radiating agent)—in other words, they either resonate or dissociate with one another. If the violin body and the bowing of the strings go together well, a relatively loud and pure sound is created that is more intense than the volume produced by plucking the strings alone.

Resonance: To co-tune; to tune a body by acting on oscillations of the same wave length (which can result in the unrestrained growth of resonance); the back-and-forth swing of electrons inside unsaturated molecules. Resonance is a phenomenon that affects all areas of our world. In physics, for example, resonance is the process by which a vibratory system is excited at its natural frequency by supplying energy. In acoustics, resonance is the reaction of two equal, identically related frequencies, from which then results a resonance frequency in which the frequencies support each other.

The formation of sound also includes the fact that there are no individual sounds in nature. Once a note is struck on the piano, played on the violin, or blown on the trumpet, all its overtones are immediately created with this single note. What we hear of these kinds of natural sound sources is always a sound that is made up of many individual tones that re-create their overtones and spread together and travel out into the world.

In a violin body, as in all resonance chambers, individual frequencies can be deleted before the sounds of these frequencies radiate out into space. The fine art of instrument making has been around for a long time; its aim is to build an instrument (a resonance chamber) with the kind of precision that deliberately deletes certain frequencies and radiates desired harmonic waves. There is the additional challenge that the sound should be perceived as alive; technically generated sounds often lack this vitality and diversity of natural tones.

It's the same with the chest and throat of a singer, which act as the resonance chamber for the vibrations of the singer's vocal cords. If the singer has an experienced voice, her sound can be so powerful that it is able to fill a concert hall without amplification, or it can even produce a sound that shatters glass. The rippling of water follows this same principle: the drop of water hits a surface—the excitation point—and the water surface then acts as a radiating veneer. A waterfall or ocean waves are manifold versions of this phenomenon.

Thus sounds generated in this natural way are fully processed by the human nervous system and the brain. This is important for our physical and mental health. A conventional speaker works due to its design, but the effects of sound produced in this mechanical way differ from a naturally produced sound in that the excitation point and the radiating surface—the speaker membrane—are identical. For this reason a conventional speaker creates a flat, two-dimensional, and direct sound, which is also much more reflective and lacks a natural quality.

TECHNICAL IMPLEMENTATION OF THE NATURSCHALLWANDLER (NATURAL SOUND TRANSDUCER)

Just like the way sound in nature radiates from one point, so does the processing of our perception need a starting point, from which we build our **listening field.** Without a clear reference point, I cannot orient myself. It's like looking at a map: if I don't know where I am, the best map is useless to me. Nature and our system of perception follow the same principle: starting from a point of excitation (the radiation point), the listening field is established.

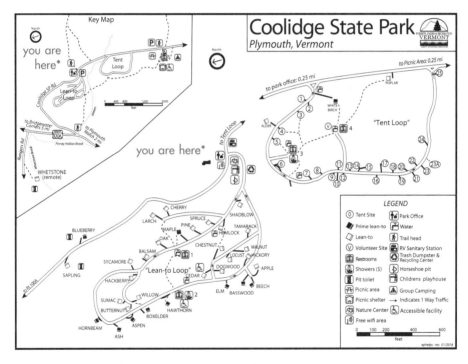

When my position is clear, I can get my bearings.

Listening field: A *field* is a region or space in which a given effect exists, therefore a listening field is the space in which we experience all the sounds of the world surrounding us through our sense of hearing. Starting from oneself as the center, all sound (or noise) is related to one particular direction. Hearing within the listening field means the ability to assign noises correctly as to from what and where they are coming.

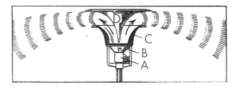

Scheme:
A) drive system
B) membrane
C) sound emitter
D) inserted funnel

Illustration by Jutta Ebinger.

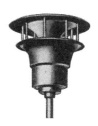

Exterior mushroom speaker made by Telefunken, from the 1930s. Image is from Der Grosse Brockhaus, Supplement 21 (Leipzig: FA Brockhaus, 1935), 515.

Where this important reference point is in humans and why it is there, I'll tell you in the next chapter. But first I want to discuss the concept of "nature-friendly" speaker technology—specifically, the Naturschallwandler natural sound transducer shown on page 39—because today this technology has become ubiquitous and has implications for how we can improve and restore human hearing naturally.

In 2003, in connection with my work in water restoration, I came across the concept of sound generation by means of Schaller speakers. This discovery came on the heels of successful pilot projects with the Senate of Berlin to explore alternative forms of improving the water quality of lakes and ponds in the city. Our remediation approach was based on using energy transmission for the biophysical restructuring of water habitats.

In 2005, I began to more intensively study the concept of using natural sound radiation to penetrate matter. Not only could this method regenerate contaminated soil and waterways, but it also soon became clear to me that the enormous effects of this natural, spherically radiating

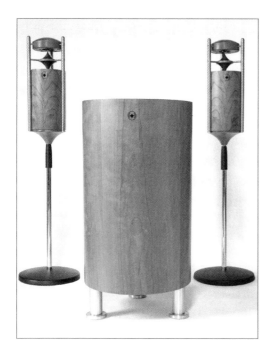

Naturschallwandler natural sound transducer (System Sunray: 2 speakers as satellites on stands and a woofer)

sound on any type of biological organism—humans in particular—could play a role in the improvement of many common hearing problems.

Over time, I was able to understand how the therapeutic application of sound works thanks to years of training and working with researchers and developers from different scientific disciplines. Specifically the areas of physics, mathematics, medicine, alternative power generation, and information technology played important contributing roles.

My own technical development of a natural sound transducer, the Naturschallwandler (NSW), reproduced nature in its perfection as realistically as possible to create an authentic sound quality, an acoustic **hologram.**

Hologram: A 3-dimensional reproduced sound that overcomes the shortcomings of monophony and stereophony, which is 1- and 2-dimensional (Greek, *holos*, "whole, complete"; and *gramma*, "weight, letter, written"). In holography, even the smallest part of a hologram contains all the information of the whole.

In doing so, the aforementioned principles of natural wave propagation had to be considered. These include:

- **The principle of omnidirectionality:** Starting from one point, a simultaneous and uniform, spherical wave propagation takes place.

- **The principle of zero pressure:** As in nature, sound waves propagate almost without pressure and evenly in three-dimensional space, overlapping harmoniously and flowing into one another without displacing one another, much like a choir singing together in which each individual voice still exists as a discrete sound.

- **The principle of resonance in space:** Without a resonance chamber and resonance body, sound cannot naturally penetrate matter. Speakers produce sound pressure regardless of their technical quality as they radiate a flat, two-dimensional direct sound. The sound pressure generated in conventional loudspeakers is neutralized by the Naturschallwandler through the creation of a precisely constructed three-dimensional geometric space. This is done by the opposite horizontal arrangement of a high- and a midrange speaker on the vertical axis and the correct placement of the **campanoid,** the core component of the Naturschallwandler, between the geometric center. The molded wooden campanoid bicone is a special geometric resonant body producing sound in the shape of a ball. Through it, the crucial point-like radiation is created.

Campanoid: A specially designed hyperbolic double cone placed between the high and middle sounder. The curve of the campanoid corresponds to the so-called Gaussian bell curve.

Natural wave radiation always connects cause or origin and space. Here, the components (for example, capacitors and inductors), the information levels (the distances of the various speakers with their characteristics relative to one another), and the areas (among other things, the geometric arrangement, the volumes of the individual body, and distances) must synchronize (coordinate the tasks of the different

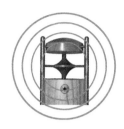

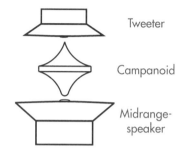

From the center of the campanoid, all frequencies of the sound can move in all directions in a space.

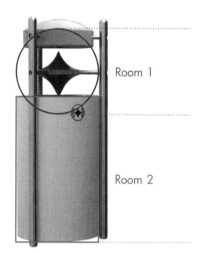

Room 1

Room 2

Tweeter

Campanoid

Midrange-speaker

Resonance-capable spatial arrangement of two-speaker information (treble center sound) in a Naturschallwandler natural sound transducer system. The tweeter and the midrange speaker create a certain frequency spectrum.

components in time) and harmonize (for example, the intensity and effects of the speakers in the room) to realize natural sound radiation technology for a total vibration that we consider pure and clear.

EXERCISE: How Well Do I Hear?

This is a simple test in 3 stages. Listening involves volume, balance, and orientation. These 3 levels build on one another in this test. You can test yourself or another person.

So far we have dealt with basic information on the sense of hearing and why strengthening our hearing is even possible. Now we want to test our current level of hearing and our reference point within the field of hearing. For this, we will use a natural sound source. A holographic speaker system like the one just mentioned can also be used if a natural sound source is insufficient for testing, as with more serious listening issues.

Listening Test with Natural Sound Source

For this test we will work with a running water tap so that we can reliably vary the volume and strength of the water jet. An indoor fountain is also suitable because it is a natural, stationary source. However, with a fountain we cannot vary the volume, which is a disadvantage, especially if we need a greater volume.

Please note that when testing with a tap we will be consuming water by letting the tap run, but in my opinion the purpose of this test justifies the use of this resource.

Preparation: Installation of a Therapeutic Listening Field

To set up the listening field, also known as the training ground, with a natural sound source, proceed as follows:

- Place a chair or stool in front of the tap. The person whose hearing is being tested, the listener, sits so that the water tap is exactly behind her back.
- Place a second chair opposite the first chair at a distance of 2 to 3 yards, facing the first chair. This is where the partner will be sitting.

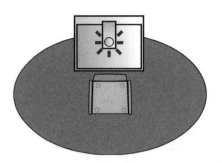

The therapeutic seating diagram with listening position in front of the tap. The listener sits with her back to the water tap.

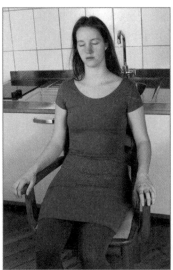

The listener with running water tap in the background

If you are testing yourself, you will need a partner to ask you various questions about your hearing perception who then records your answers as well as their own observations. The partner will be sitting in the second chair. Give yourselves enough time for the entire test.

Note to Hearing Aid Users

The determination of the listener's current hearing status is best carried out without a hearing aid. With a fair amount of hearing loss, depending on the degree of loss, the exercise should be explained in detail and should, if needed, include an agreed-upon hand signal for volume control prior to the removal of the hearing aid. If the person being tested cannot understand anything without wearing the hearing aid, even very loud speaking, then the entire test should be performed with the hearing aid. In such a case the training should proceed according to the instructions in this book, but over a longer period of time, before trying to continue the work again without a hearing aid. The amount of time needed for training will depend on individual needs.

1st Stage: Determination of General Hearing

Now the test can begin. Follow all the steps in order:

- The listener sits relaxed and comfortable in the training seat. The partner sits opposite her on the second chair with pen and paper ready to record his observations and the listener's answers to questions. The faucet is still off.
- The partner asks the listener to close her eyes, then he quietly goes to the faucet and slowly turns it on so that only a small, steady stream comes out of the tap.
- The partner goes back to the chair across from the listener, sits down, and asks, "Can you clearly hear the sound of water?"
- If the listener is unable to hear the sound of the water clearly, the

faucet is turned up in stages so that gradually more and more water is flowing. To do this, the partner goes to the faucet to open it further and then goes back to the chair opposite the listener, once again asking if she can hear clearly. Proceeding this way, the water faucet is turned up successively in stages until the listener can clearly hear the sound of the running water.

- For those who are more hard of hearing, you can increase the volume by placing a pot right side up or upside down under the faucet, or you can use something else with a tinny sound when struck by water. Make sure your modifications are suitable to amplify the sound of the running water, and have them ready to implement.
- Once you've reached a volume that is heard well by the listener, compare this volume with that of a normal conversation. If the water noise is louder, this indicates a weakness in the listener's hearing.

2nd Stage: Testing the Balance of the Right/Left Auditory Field

This is a test of whether we hear equally well with both ears. Proceed step-by-step:

- The faucet is still running at the volume the listener can discern.
- The listener remains relaxed, sitting with eyes closed.
- The partner sits in the chair opposite, looks at the listener, and checks the following:
  - ► What is the position of her head?
  - ► Is her head straight?
  - ► Is her head is rotated and/or held at an angle?
  - ► Are her shoulders about the same height?

Use the blank diagram shown as a guide to draw the position of the axes of the listener, checking her head and shoulder positions.

Note that different strengths between the left and right auditory perception or a unilateral hearing loss are almost always reflected in a

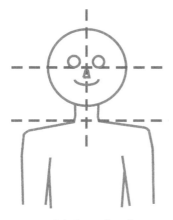

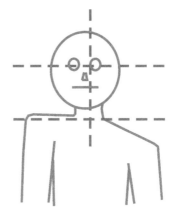

A balanced and symmetrical figure

An out-of-balance figure

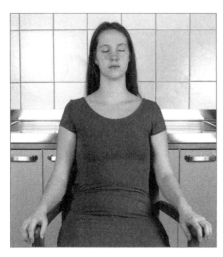

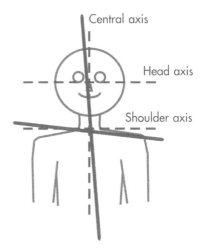

The person with a slight shift: the left shoulder of the person in the diagram is slightly deeper than the right, while the head is tilted slightly to the right.

Out-of-balance axes in the sketch of the person seated in the photograph

more or less unbalanced posture and **body geometry** in the vertical and horizontal planes. In such a case a specific ear is usually rotated forward; this is usually the stronger ear. In general, if the head is not directed straight forward, this is considered a very strong indication that one ear is stronger than the other. This relationship of imbalance and hearing will be further explored in the next stage of this test.

Body geometry: The balance and symmetry of the body in the vertical and horizontal planes

3rd Stage: Orientation/Location of the Sound Source

This part of the test is about the ability to correctly locate a sound source in a space without an optical reference. Proceed step-by-step:

- Once the listener is seated and relaxed and has been listening to the splashing sound of the water for a while, the partner asks, "Where do you hear the sound of the water coming from? Please indicate with your hand." It is important that the person actually points to the location of the sound and doesn't just describe the location. This physical gesture increases perception and makes the hearing situation clearer.

- If the location is not clear to the listener, the partner repeats this question once or twice, waiting for a short period of time between asking until the sound is clearly indicated by the listener. Crucial to this question is whether the listener *actually* hears the sound, no matter where it's coming from to her, and not where she *thinks* the sound is coming from. We need to establish this starting point of perceptual orientation for further training. It may be that the noise of the water "moves" from the listener's perception; that is, it is perceived during the course of testing as being in different positions in the room. This is actually a good sign and shows that the hearing system in the person works because it is seeking order. Allow the listener some time in this case. However, if at this point in the test it's not possible for the listener to clearly locate the water noise after 1 to 2 minutes, leave it at that and conclude the test.

- If the water noise is heard as coming from any different position in the room than the correct height, which depends on where the water jet hits (for example, above or diagonally behind the listener), then the acoustic localization has not yet been adjusted.

The partner notes where the listener hears the sound of running water coming from by means of a diagram, as shown on page 47.

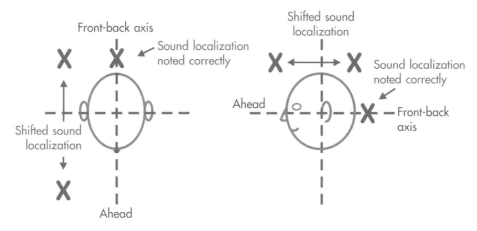

Determining the position of water noise in the listening field

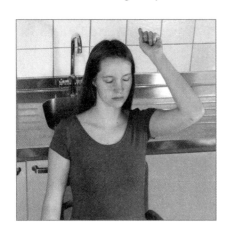

The listener shows where she hears the sound of running water coming from. Here she hears the noise source shifted to her left and too high from the correct location.

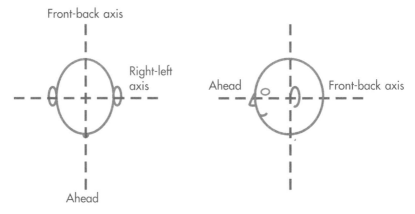

A blank template for determining the position of the sound of running water in a listening field

Use the blank template at the bottom of page 47 to record the perceived position of water noise. Note that for a correct acoustic localization, the listener should hear the sound of water coming from behind her, exactly in the middle of her orientation, and at the correct height.

Terminating the Listening Test

Once you get to the end of the test, slowly and gradually turn off the water until it is no longer running. Tell the listener that she can slowly open her eyes again. Give her some time before discussing the results.

Conclusion and Debriefing

Although the test outlined here does have a training effect in that it prepares the listener for the training to come, it is primarily an important initial inventory of the person's current hearing/listening status.

Next, both parties will discuss the results of this test and any observations in an open and sensitive manner. Each of you should share your perceptions of what you saw and experienced at each of the 3 stages of the test. This discussion is not about being fixated on results; we have merely identified the status of the listener's hearing. Most important, these results are not immutable facts. It must also be noted that many people do not even realize that they have a hearing deficiency, or how bad it is.

So, what next? You'll find out in chapter 2, Return to the Center. Below I describe the first variant of the hearing test with the Naturschallwandler natural sound transducer, which is helpful to use if a natural sound source is insufficient for testing, as with more serious listening issues.

Listening Test with the Naturschallwandler Natural Sound Transducer

This test is done in 3 stages. You will need an amplifier with a remote control, a CD player or other audio source, and a natural sound transducer system such as the Naturschallwandler. The test will not work with conventional speakers. Convenient but not essential is a decibel display of the music system.

Preparation: Installation of a Therapeutic Listening Field

To set up the listening field with the Naturschallwandler natural sound transducer system, proceed as follows:

- Set up the system in front of a wall and connect it in accordance with the assembly instructions. Make sure that both speakers are the same distance from the therapeutic chair you'll be using, as shown in the figure below.
- Set the 2 speakers on stands at the lowest height so that the campanoid is located approximately at heart level when the listener is seated.
- Place a sturdy chair (such as a stable wicker chair) or stool exactly in the middle between the two speakers. This is the therapeutic seat where the listener will be sitting.
- Place the bass module left or right between the chair and the speakers or, more optimally, directly behind the seat.
- If possible, place the chair directly against the wall, or if the bass module is behind the chair, place it a few centimeters in front of the module. This arrangement of the therapeutic seat can also take

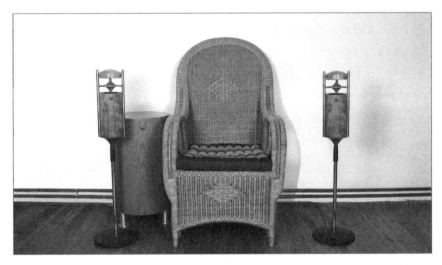

Therapeutic listening position with Naturschallwandler natural sound transducer

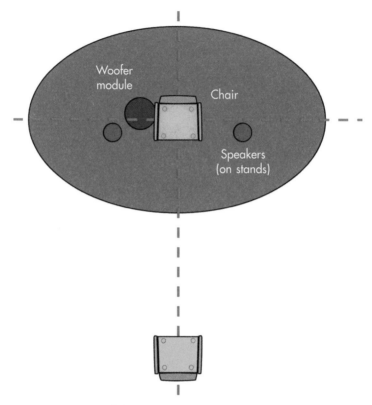

Arrangement of the therapeutic listening field in plane view

place in the middle of a room; however, it is easier for the listener to sit directly against a wall, as this orientation to the wall tends to give the person a feeling of security.

- The speakers and the upper body of the person sitting in the chair should be aligned.
- Set up a second chair opposite the therapeutic seat at a distance of 2 to 3 yards for monitoring. This chair is for the partner.

Musical Requirements

You will need a song featuring a single female singer, that is, vocals with a simple musical accompaniment, with the following qualities:

- The voice of the singer must be centered—that is, equal distance from the speakers of the Naturschallwandler natural sound transducer and the middle position of the balance control of the amplifier—so that the singer can be heard exactly in the middle.

- The song should have dynamics—that is, different volumes—and should be sung in several pitches.

- The song should have pleasant content. Just take one that pleases you and makes you feel good. These requirements are fulfilled by the song "Over the Rainbow" by Eva Cassidy (from her album *Songbird*). We've been using this song with great success for many years now.

You will be working in pairs, same as in the previous test. The partner will be asking the listener questions about her hearing perception and will record her answers and make observations. Allow time for this process. The test song can be repeated once or twice until all test questions have been answered. The person being tested should have an opportunity to tune in to the music and experience holographic listening.

Now the test with the natural sound transducers can begin.

Note to Hearing Aid Users

The determination of the listener's current hearing status is best carried out without a hearing aid. With a fair amount of hearing loss, depending on the degree of loss, the exercise should be explained in detail and should, if needed, include agreed-upon hand signals including one for volume control prior to the removal of the hearing aid. If the person being tested cannot understand anything without wearing the hearing aid, even very loud speaking, then the entire test should be performed with the hearing aid in place. In such a case the training should proceed according to the instructions in this book over a longer period of time before trying to continue again without a hearing aid. The amount of time needed for training will depend on individual needs.

1st Stage: Detecting General Hearing in Conjunction with Volume

Proceed step-by-step as follows:

- The listener sits relaxed and comfortable in the training chair. The partner sits down in the chair across from her and holds the remote control, as well as a pen and paper to record important observations and the listener's answers to questions.
- The partner asks the listener to close her eyes.
- The partner now plays the selected song, starting out softly, at a low volume, and then slowly and gradually turning up the volume until the singer's voice is heard clearly by the listener. The partner finds this out by asking: 1) "Is the volume pleasant?" and 2) "Can you hear the singer well?" These questions are repeated each time the volume is adjusted until the listener can affirm both questions. (Note that if you use Eva Cassidy's rendition of "Over the Rainbow" as your selection, there is an instrumental part in the middle of the song, so wait through that section of music.)
- Comparing the volume of the song to the volume of a voice in a normal spoken conversation gives us an indication of what the general state of the listener's hearing is at this time. If the volume needs to be louder before the listener hears the song as pleasant, this indicates a weakness in hearing.

2nd Stage: Testing the Balance of the Right/Left Auditory Field

This is a test of whether we hear equally well with both ears. Proceed step-by-step:

- The music continues as before, at the level the listener can discern, while the listener remains seated and relaxed, with eyes closed.
- The partner looks at the listener and checks:
  - ▶ What is the position of her head?
  - ▶ Is her head straight?
  - ▶ Is her head rotated and/or held at an angle?

▶ Are her shoulders even, at about the same height?

Use the diagram below on the left as a template to draw the position of the axes of the listener.

Comments and hints: A different strength between the left and the right auditory perception or a unilateral hearing loss is almost always reflected in a more or less unbalanced body posture and geometry.

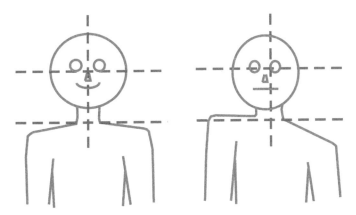

The listener on the left is balanced and symmetrical. The listener on the right is unbalanced (which indicates an imbalance in hearing).

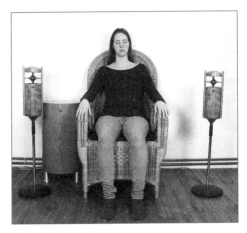

The listener with the Naturschallwandler (natural sound transducer) system. Her upper body axes show a slight shift, with the her right shoulder a little deeper than the left, and the head tilted slightly to her right.

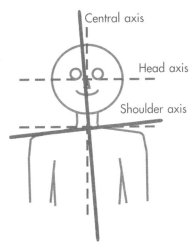

Central axis

Head axis

Shoulder axis

The alignment of axes in the person photographed transferred to a diagram

In particular, if an ear is rotated forward, this is usually the stronger ear. In other words, if the head is not directed straight forward, this is considered a strong indication that the listening field of one side is stronger than the other. This relationship of posture imbalance and hearing will be further investigated in the 3rd stage of this test.

3rd Stage: Orientation/Location of the Sound Source

This part of the test is about the ability to correctly locate a sound source in space without an optical reference. Proceed step-by-step:

- After the listener has been relaxed and listening to the song for a while, the partner asks, "Where do you hear the singer? Please indicate with your hand." It is important that the listener gestures with her hand and does not simply describe where she hears the singer. This body action makes the existing hearing situation clear.

- If this question cannot be answered by the listener at first, the partner repeats the question 1 or 2 more times, with a time interval in between, until the singer is heard clearly. The decisive factor is where the person *actually* hears the singer. It is not important to hear the singer at the "right" place; it is not about "knowing" where the sound is coming from but rather where the person actually hears the voice coming from, no matter where that location is. We need this starting point for further training.

- It may be that the listener perceives the singer as "moving" over a period of time, as though hearing from different positions in the room. This is a good sign and shows that the hearing of the person is working because it is seeking order.

   Give the person some time in this case. As explained at the beginning of the test description, the song can be repeated if all the steps do not yield clear-cut answers. If no clear localization is possible at this point of the test after 2 to 3 minutes, leave it at that and conclude the test.

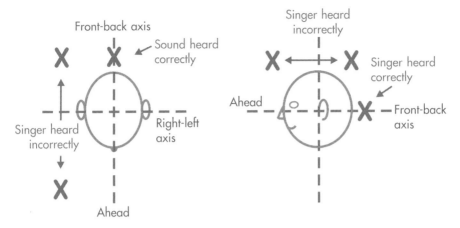

Determining the position of the singer's voice in the room

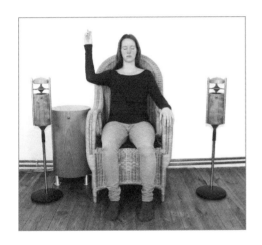

The listener shows where she hears the singer's voice coming from. Here she hears the singer's voice coming from her right and too high.

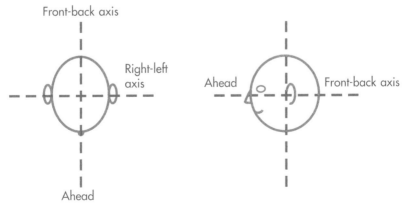

Blank template for determining the position of the singer's voice in the room

■ If the singer is heard in a different position in the room other than in the area behind the listener's head—for example, above, in front, or angled from the rear—the acoustic location has not yet adjusted. That's no problem, as we have training and detailed instructions for correcting this later in this book.

Following your observations of where the person hears the singer's voice coming from, you will note that information in a diagram, using the blank template provided on the bottom of page 55. In a correct acoustic alignment the listener will hear the singer's voice at the back of her head, ideally right in the middle.

Terminating the Listening Test

As the song plays begin adjusting the volume gradually so that the sound gets quieter and quieter until it is no longer heard. Once you have arrived at the end of the song, turn off the recording. Tell the listener to slowly open her eyes. Give her some time before you start to discuss the results.

Conclusion and Debriefing

Although this preliminary test has a training effect, it is primarily an inventory of the listener's hearing. Discuss the results and observations with each other in a sensitive manner. As a partner, discuss your observations at each stage. The listener too should discuss what she experienced. This is not about fixating on results. We are examining the listener's current hearing status. This is not an immutable situation, and in fact many people don't even realize that they have a hearing deficit or how bad their hearing really is.

In this chapter we have gone through 2 tests measuring 3 levels of hearing. In the 2nd and 3rd stages of the tests we focused on perception of a centerpoint and the associated ability to build symmetry. Now we will explore these matters in greater detail.

2

Return to the Center

*Balancing the Body to Self-Regulate
Orientation and Hearing*

BALANCE IS A PRINCIPLE of all holistic systems of health and healing. To have balance we must arrive at the center. I don't mean this in a spiritual sense—even though awareness of the center does have a spiritual aspect—I am talking about a concrete, physical sensation. In martial arts, yoga, qigong, and similar modalities, this center is perceived as being two finger widths below the navel and is referred to as the *hara*. To move from this center and to breathe from there strengthens our steadfastness and balances us. Balancing results in gentle and flowing emotions that can make our perceptions clear and the control of our body easier. If I'm physically out of balance, my body will need more energy than when I move from my center.

In this chapter we will explore balance and why it is so crucial to our listening and our hearing. Meanwhile, here's a great exercise to explore your center.

(( ) EXERCISE: Flying across a Meadow with Arms Outstretched

Remember how you "flew" as a child, with arms outstretched, racing across a field or meadow? Try it. Follow your gut feelings and the speed that feels good. Try flapping your "wings" if you like.

Comments and hints: This movement stimulates the entire body and strengthens your sense of balance. Hold your head up high and look to the horizon. Gently rock your torso back and forth, tilting from one side to another as you fly. This complex sequence of movements specifically strengthens the back muscles in the process of allowing your body to naturally find its center.

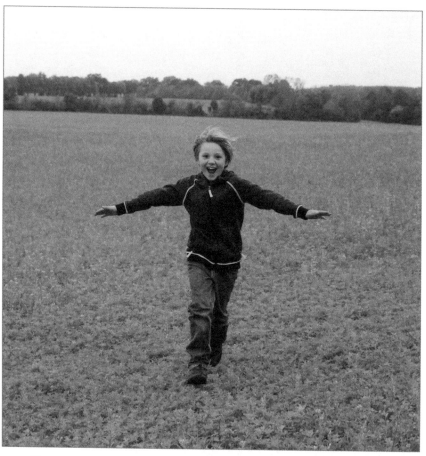

Flying across a meadow like a child strengthens our sense of balance.
Photo by Mara Ebinger.

HUMAN CONSCIOUSNESS AND HEARING

Hearing consists of two equal, dynamic processes that occur simultaneously and constantly interact with each other in synchronous and equivalent ways. Both processes are in direct communication with our consciousness; that is, that aspect of ourselves that perceives itself and says, "I am."

Consciousness has 2 aspects. One consists of the sum of all things of which I am aware, which I call my memory. The other aspect is what is understood as the subconsciousness, mental activities just below the threshold of awareness, those aspects of awareness that are not immediately accessible to the conscious mind yet are still there; for example, experiences I've forgotten but that I can be made aware of again through various mental and physical processes, like attempting to find an object I've misplaced by trying to remember the last time I was in contact with it and actively searching for it in that place. Our consciousness processes perception, always confronting both dynamic hearing processes, which are:

- **Hearing threshold and identification:** What's being said? What is the information being transmitted? How do I interpret a sound if I can barely hear it because the volume is beyond my threshold of perception?
- **Location and individual assignment:** Where does the noise come from? Where is the source of the noise in the room?

"Ah, there's a car!" Hearing it is one thing. However, how does it move in relation to me? Without this information, the auditory perception of the car isn't of much use to me. It possibly puts pressure on me because deep down inside I know: *Car—watch out! It could run me over.* That means that I have to be attentive. It's a potential danger I likely learned about early in life as a child. Depending on the experiences I've had with cars, my conscious attention is now joined by my subconscious awareness that constantly perceives and analyzes my environment. This

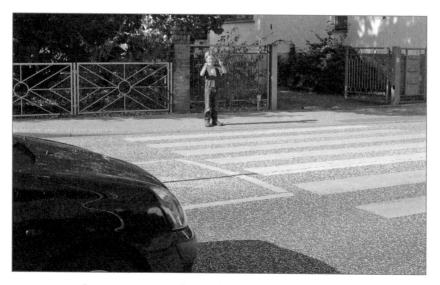

Perceiving a noise that could potentially cause danger.
Photo by Mara Ebinger.

is the individual assignment of sound. If we have no "experience space" for a certain sound, we must learn its associations as soon as possible. Parents know this and therefore pay close attention to their children who are learning to assess danger and acting accordingly.

This individual assessment of my localization/current situation is quite an important point when it comes to hearing. We can only be aware of a sound and its associations if we've perceived that sound (i.e., heard it) and located its source. In this example, "car" means, among other things, potential danger, especially if I'm in the street as one approaches. In earlier times, when a hungry bear growled in the forest, it was good to know from which direction it was growling. Then you could choose where and how you wanted to react—most likely running as far away from that sound as possible.

HEARING IS A LEARNING PROCESS

Human evolution gives the ear primary importance even in the embryo state, because it is the first developed organ of perception. In the brain, a strikingly large space is reserved for listening. This doesn't only include hearing sounds, it also involves perceiving sound frequencies (the number of oscillations in the form of waves) and sound forms and internally reacting to them. Even unborn children react joyfully when their parents talk to them. All living organisms, not just humans, have this initial possibility of perception through sound waves and vibrations.

Nature has perfectly equipped us with a three-dimensional sense of hearing to perceive, sense, and feel the world around us. Listening is a key area of perception, our existential connection to the world. If we look with our eyes, we are going outside of ourselves. When we hear, we take the external world inside of us and feel and sense how this affects us, which is resonance. The result is a permanently existing, ongoing interaction (in the background) between the person and his or her living environment. In listening, we determine whether we should be active or at rest, and whether something is near or far, familiar or foreign, a threat or a haven. The power, dynamic, and emotion of each source of noise is detected and placed in our consciousness, where it is assigned diverse meanings. For example, do I hear a friendly or a hostile voice?

Human beings always seek their position in relation to surrounding situations on all levels of perception: body, mind, and soul. Where am *I*? What is around *me*? What is *my* relationship (proximity, distance, size, etc.) to my environment? Spatial perception is primarily controlled by the eyes and ears, which are responsible for different aspects of spatial orientation. The eyes are directed to the front, and to a limited extent to the sides, and serve to focus on objects in our surroundings and to spatially distinguish them from one another. The field of vision of the eyes is about 120 degrees, so they are primarily used for orientation to the front half of our world. Our ears are different: With them we can perceive impressions from 360 degrees around us. They serve the full spatial orientation in all directions. And not only that, but we can also perceive events with our ears when we cannot see them directly or they are far away; for example, a siren, an approaching thunderstorm, a dog barking next door, or children's laughter in the next room.

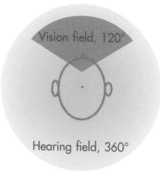

The hearing field informs us from all directions.

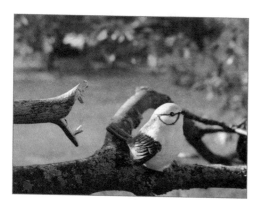

Do I hear a snake behind me, or is it the rustling of a bird in the tree?

Thus listening is very closely related to our ability to assess, perceive, and intuitively interpret danger. To hear what's happening behind you is of fundamental importance.

If parts of our sensory apparatus are limited or completely diminished, the remaining senses become more important. For example, a blind person is particularly dependent on hearing as a vital source of information about their surroundings—just as a sighted person would be in complete darkness. Their hearing is so sharp and trained so perfectly that their orientation takes place almost exclusively in an acoustic way. If a sighted man walks on the sidewalk and hears an approaching cyclist from behind who wants to pass him, he reflexively turns to find out where the cyclist is located. Only then does he decide if and where he'll dodge the cyclist. He reflexively uses his eyes to clarify the situation, although with good hearing this may not be necessary. All too often he does not rely on his sense of hearing. The blind man, however, is able to correctly detect the cyclist based on acoustic perception of the cyclist's movement and location, and he easily gets out of the way. If the blind man accidentally drops a coin from his wallet on the floor, he can correctly guess its location based on the sound of the impact and can then pick up the coin. The blind man is able to create an accurate three-dimensional localization and mapping of objects in space because of the noise that was generated when the coin hit the floor. He has optimally trained his sense of hearing as a result of his lack of vision and uses it in daily life to ensure independence and survival.

LOCATING THE SOURCE OF SOUND FROM A REFERENCE POINT

The processing and spatial orientation of a sound source needs a reference point from which we build and calculate our listening field. The reference point allows us to record, process, and classify sound. We need it as a starting point for spatial processing, and it is fundamentally important for the allocation of all information. In terms of hearing, this reference point is the area that lies at the back of the head.

We need to identify and classify the information we hear. The more complete the information we receive, the easier it is to process. The more precisely our internal system is arranged, the more comprehensively we can process our perceptions of the external world—and the stronger and deeper is our capacity for self-regulation. When we can locate sound spatially we simply hear better.

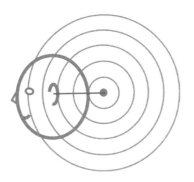

The reference point for the configuration of the listening field is centered in the area behind the head.

There is always a specific cause for a hearing problem: it is usually associated with a stressful acoustic event that one experienced at some point in life. I don't mean trauma in a purely mechanical sense, as in interlocking gears where if I stop one, the whole machine stands still. Rather, I refer to this in a **cybernetic** sense, meaning a change, a weakening, a violation of a part as a result of an acoustic incident, which leads to a change in the whole system. When this trauma causes us to lose our ability to locate sound spatially, we must also work on processing the traumatic experience. The more we are able to process the traumatic experience, the better our ability to locate sound becomes, and the better we are able to hear again.

> **Cybernetics:** A science that deals with the control and regulation of a wide variety of natural and artificial systems, in particular, the recording, processing, and transmission of examined information (Greek, *kybernetike*, "pilot, governor"); the science of communication and control theory that is concerned with the comparative study of automatic control systems such as the nervous system and the brain

EXERCISE: Hearing Someone from Behind

Have someone stand behind you at a distance of about 2 yards. She speaks a few sentences, but so quietly that you can barely hear her. By listening, try to determine:

- Where is she?
- Is she of the same height as you? If so, then you should also be able to locate her voice exactly from behind at an appropriate distance, at about the level of the back of your head.
- If she is smaller or taller than you, the correct location of her voice will be slightly below or above the back of your head.
- Now make a note where you have actually heard her voice.

Comments and hints: This exercise is not about doing it "right," it's about strengthening your sound-locating ability. Particularly, if you have weak hearing, if you cannot hear certain frequencies, if you listen one-sidedly, if you have difficulty locating the sound source, if you have spatial disorientation while listening to multiple sound sources, then the perceived location of the sound source differs significantly from the center of the front-back axis. In this exercise, sometimes a person will locate the person behind them but away from the reference point. Sometimes a person will turn their head to locate the source of sound from behind, so they are compensating with their body for a perception deficit in which the location of the sound is not precisely known. In this case the person can no longer hear in a relaxed fashion—he has lost his ability to correctly locate sound sources and therefore has lost order in his system. (The training to build up correct positioning is explained in chapter 5). The consequences of these kinds of deficits in sound locating are that our ability to process information slows down with the stress of trying compensate for the weakness, and our body coordination and fine motor skills lose their precision with the effort of trying to locate the source of the sound. This exercise can be repeated often to train your sense of listening to a sound source that is behind you.

THE REFERENCE POINT

The aim of the basic method of hearing regeneration is to rebuild the original order of acoustic perception. This is a prerequisite to regenerating hearing. We know that nothing regrows in the ear anatomically, so for change to occur the brain must learn to process existing information optimally and completely. Hearing is not just about mechanics, it is the result of the interplay of the ear itself, the nervous system, and the brain. It takes time to counteract situations that for years and decades have placed burdens on us and caused changes in us. And so hearing regeneration is about building one's ability to self-regulate through proper physiological training. For example, when I begin to train my muscles correctly at the gym, they become stronger. It's the same way for hearing, it just involves a different set of "muscles."

Let's return to the subject of a reference point, which in the case of hearing lies in the area immediately at the back of the head. Here, the brain, in conjunction with the ears, calculates the location of all sources of sound in the listening field. Using this area behind the head as a reference point, an equilateral triangle is formed with the two ears, which defines this reference point. If this triangle were to shift more to the right or to the left, or up or down, then I would not have a symmetrical reference system for the sound waves to hit my ears. This means my system cannot accurately calculate the location of the sound source, and this makes hearing difficult, especially when multiple sound sources are occurring simultaneously.

If we don't have a reliable reference point our system will attempt to create it, constantly calculating and adjusting. This is one of the reasons why we sometimes hear badly, which also depends on what kind of day we are having. This is also why at times it may take longer to process specific acoustic information. If that only happens once in a while, we can deal with it. However, as a permanent condition it can lead to stress, tension, and uncertainty: "I feel burdened by having to listen so hard." If it's too difficult to hear, we stop trying and tune out.

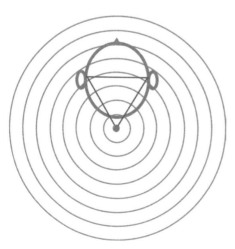

The configuration of the listening field using the triangular reference point formed by the two ears and the space immediately behind the head, the reference point

THE BODY'S REACTIONS TO STRESS

When we're under stress, our entire system reacts. As soon as possible it will seek to process the burden and rebalance itself. Our bodies naturally want to return quickly to equilibrium and a relaxed state.

For many people, listening has become a burden due to stress. Stress can come in many forms: the persistent sound of a loud, dissonant jackhammer at a construction site; the continuous background noise in big cities, where even at night no natural silence comes; and even the emotional and mental stress of constant arguing and having to listen to words you do not want to hear.

Natural harmonic sounds are literally food for the brain and the soul because they stimulate our gray matter. It has been found that listening to a piano concerto—if we enjoy that kind of music—can improve our "visual-spatial efficiency," a phenomenon called the "Mozart effect."[1] Natural harmonic sounds affect our body through their rhythm. When we perceive the soothing, melodic song of a nightingale, our own rhythm entrains with the bird's song as our heartbeat aligns with it. If, on the other hand, we are constantly exposed to highway or aircraft noise, these disharmonious sounds lead to an unnatural rhythm that weakens us physically, emotionally, and mentally.

Stress can also occur when I cannot correctly locate a sound. Say I hear a sound from a human or a car and I have to check with my eyes to see where it's coming from. If I find that it does not come from where I thought I had heard it coming from, or if I did not even hear the sound and then suddenly I see its cause, such as an approaching car, I get scared and become unsure.

Listening always involves perception and the process of internally re-creating an authentic image of what we glean from the outside. As well, hearing involves more than just superficial content. For example, we determine whether a statement is true or false based on a feeling related to the nuance of hearing what is being said between the lines of what is being conveyed in words.

Listening when experiencing stress and uncertainty can cause the body to react in various ways, depending on the stressor, including:

- Release of adrenaline
- Disorientation
- Confusion up to paralysis
- Tension and increased stress levels

If we don't reduce our stress level, we'll feel exhausted, we can't sleep, and when we finally do fall asleep we don't feel rested in the morning.

All these are symptoms of having lost our center, our homeostasis. The ability of our integrated system to self-regulate and regenerate is thus impaired because we can only regenerate when we're relaxed. Long-term, this leads to burnout, which basically describes the condition of exhaustion in which our entire organism is overloaded—a condition in earlier times that was called *cachexia,* "wasting disease," or malnutrition. In modern times this condition supposedly doesn't exist, although chronic stress can bring about the same results.

LET'S TAKE A LOOK IN THE MIRROR

Balance and equilibrium are basic features of a healthy system and an important support for the body's regulatory processes. Whether we feel safe and comfortable is also determined by how well-balanced we are on the purely physical plane. We can explore our balance by doing this exercise:

EXERCISE: Bending Back and Forth

Follow these step-by-step instructions:

- Stand upright and relaxed.
- Bend slightly forward and feel that even this slight shift from your center requires additional effort so that you don't fall over.
- Take a few steps in this position. For this, you will need even more effort.

- Increase the amount of effort you will need by carefully taking a few steps backward in the same position. The feeling of insecurity continues to intensify.

Comments and hints: At the beginning of this exercise, when you're upright, there is a natural sense of balance with the concurrent ability to relax in this position because of the physical conditions on this planet. Gravity is the force that allows us to stay upright and centered and relaxed at the same time. The more I deviate from this natural order, the more resistance to the center I create. In the upright position there is less energy expended and more opportunities for movement. Movement from one's center is effortless, lighter, and more relaxed.

To stay in balance we need direction and focus. Direction is maintained by Earth's gravitational force pulling downward. In outer space there is no balance because gravity is absent. Our body's equillibrium and our mental balance is in a static state when we stand and don't move. When we move these become dynamic and are maintained along 4 main horizontal axes and 1 vertical central axis (see page 70).

We have in these axes a symmetry; that is, a balance, for complete awareness and control of our bodies. The basic structure of the human organism (as well as most other organisms) is based on **bilateral** symmetry: 2 eyes to see in 3 dimensions; 2 ears to hear in 3 dimensions, and so on. Cognition depends on that symmetry. Without it, I don't feel like I'm in control. Since hearing is closely linked to body geometry and bilateral symmetry, you can improve upon those physical capabilities by doing the exercise on pages 70–75.

Bilateral: Two-sided, so that one plane divides the individual into essentially two identical halves; related to or affecting the right and left sides of the body or the right and left members of paired organs (Latin, *bi,* "two"; and *lateralis,* "side")

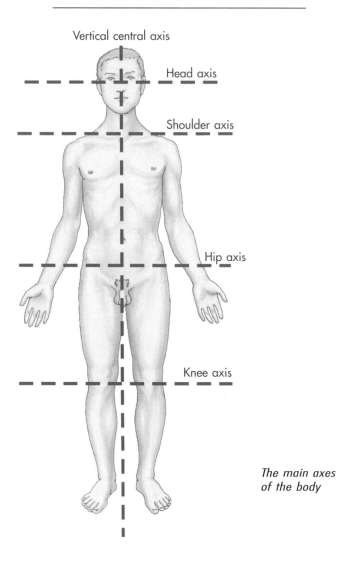

Vertical central axis

Head axis

Shoulder axis

Hip axis

Knee axis

*The main axes
of the body*

EXERCISE: Working with a Mirror

Do this exercise with a mirror in which you can see at least your head
and shoulder area. The mirror must hang vertically so that the image
is not distorted. Follow the directions step-by-step and see photos on
pages 72–75.

- Sit or stand in front of the mirror.
- Now close your eyes.

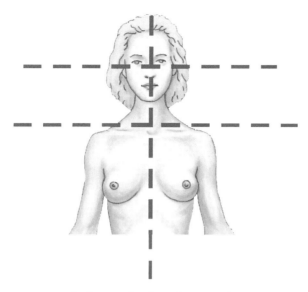

Body axes for the mirror exercise

- Assume a comfortable position with your hands by your side.
- Take a few relaxed breaths.
- Align yourself in front of the mirror by concentrating on your head and shoulders so that they feel straight and centered.
- Now open your eyes and observe how your body geometry is aligned with respect to the head and shoulder axis, including the spacing of the arms to the body.
- With your eyes still open, pay special attention to the orientation of your head, centering it along the vertical axis, including the distance of your arms from your body.
- With your eyes still open, correct the position of your shoulders, relaxing the higher-lying shoulder until it is level with the lower-lying shoulder. If aligning your shoulders is difficult or impossible, relax and balance your shoulders to whatever extent possible.
- Now close your eyes again and breathe in and out slowly. As you inhale, bring your hands to your chest, palms facing upward, as if lifting something up.
- When your hands reach the upper body, turn the palms inward.

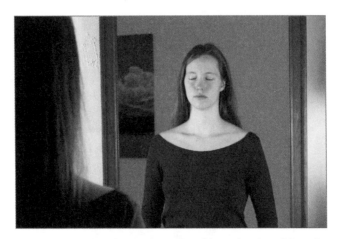

With your eyes closed, stand comfortably with relaxed breathing.

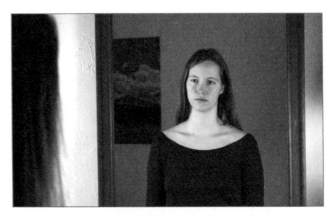

Open your eyes and observe your body axes.

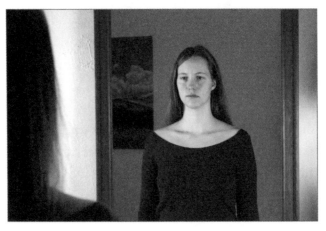

With eyes open, align the head and shoulder axes.

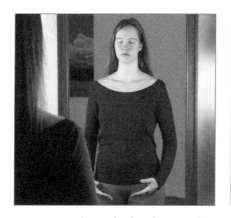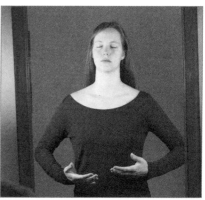

Begin to bring the hands toward your chest, palms up.

"Open" your hands, palms upward, as if you're lifting something.

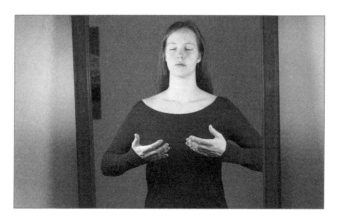

At the upper body, the hands turn inward.

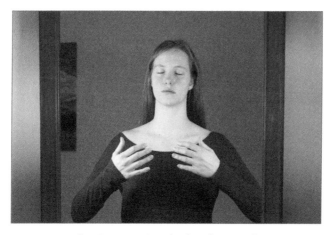

Continue turning the hands inward.

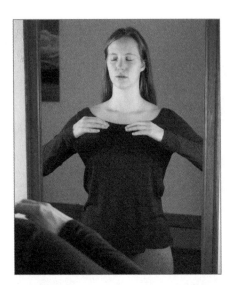

Exhale, and begin to guide the palms downward.

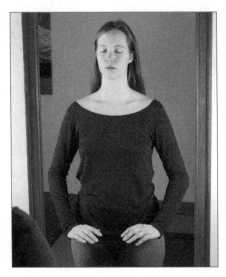

Lower the hands with palms facing downward.

- As you breathe out, guide your open palms downward and let them relax palms-down in front of the body, as shown above.
- Relax your arms and hands, resting them lightly on the front of your body, palms facing down.
- Open your eyes. Try this exercise a few times.

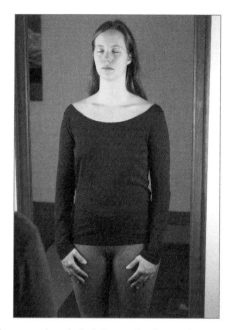

Relax your hands lightly on the front of your body.
This is the end of the exercise.

Comments and hints: This seemingly simple exercise has its challenges. If you correct your body with your eyes, you may notice that what you feel as "straight" is actually completely crooked. By doing the exercise daily, the body will begin to realign itself and balance over time. Be patient, because changes in body geometry take time as muscles, joints, and joint positions change. It may even happen that your body will feel uncomfortable at one point or another because over time the regulation process releases deeper tensions.

The mirror exercise allows you to create a reference point to the Earth by using the force of gravity to help you align. This reference point provides safety and security for your body. When I don't feel secure in my own body I cannot self-regulate because I cannot relax. That's why I have to build a sense of security in my body and the feeling of having both feet firmly on the ground.

Again, as always, follow your feelings as you do this exercise, and don't overextend yourself. Respect your limits. Do not force yourself to hold a straight posture, because by doing so you are forcing a desire. Do not skip any steps in the exercise, the purpose of which is to bring the inner feeling of "straightness" in line with the external visible reality. Your perception of your physical being is what's crucial here. The mirror exercise is not about end results but about starting a process. The hand movements and breathing help your body, over time, to acquire the ability to remember what straight and centered feels like.

3

Our Desire to Hear and Feel

Our Ears Connect Us to the World

In the great ancient civilizations, not the eye, but the ear was considered our noblest sense. "The ear is the way" it says in the Upanishads, the registry of Indian wisdom.

J. E. BERENDT

SOUND IS ALWAYS PRESENT. Something audible is continuously happening all around us. We constantly hear, whether or not we like it. The ear cannot close naturally; it has no lid, no muscle, no reflex that could consciously create a barrier between our acoustic perception and the outside world. We listen to sounds from the start of life and for the duration of our entire life.

The world of the audible is infinitely diverse: it includes a **myriad** of unique sound and frequency patterns that can vary from total chaos to complete order, from almost indefinable noise and sound shreds, to aesthetically pleasing, exhilarating, highly complex sound shapes and structures, such as music and singing.

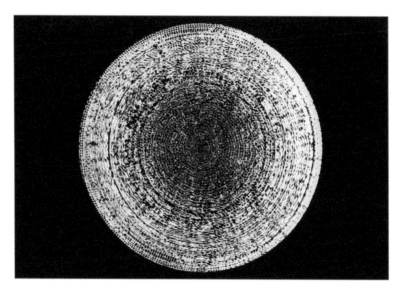

Water sound image. Water—here in a glass dish—absorbs the vibrations of sounds and forms depending on the type of sound, which can be seen with the right kind of lighting that shows a special pattern. Photo by Alexander Lauterwasser from his book Wasser, Klang, Bilder *(AT Verlag: Aarau, 2002).*

Myriad: 10,000; a great number or quantity (Greek, *myrias*, the number "10,000")

All around us is an often unnoticed acoustic cosmos that is constantly re-creating itself, expressing and communicating all the evolutionary processes in a buzzing and resonant way. The entire universe is filled with sounds, waves, and vibrations. Astronomers can measure cosmic background noise coming from all directions.

The development of language in its diverse and numerous sounds and melodies is a fundamental acoustic pillar of human culture. Without listening and fully understanding, the individual human being as well as human civilization can neither rise nor permanently survive in a healthy manner. It is written in the Bible, "In the beginning was the Word." And the word finds its form through sound: vibration and harmony, frequency and timbre, rhythm and timing, volume and content determine how we record acoustic information.

Then God said, "Let there be light!" That's what the book of Genesis says. In all religions, Creation begins with the transformation of the idea (spirit) into form (matter) by means of vibration. Human language, including the language of the Creation event or the language of God, is shaped by syllables that have the potential to shape matter itself. We share the world through language, thoughts, and related feelings. We put into words what we want, what we need, what should happen, and what should be carried out. Connected is our feeling of empowerment, self-determination, and freedom, or on the other hand, impotence. Can we shape the world as we want it? Can we express ourselves? Can we share? Can we understand ourselves and the world around us? It all begins with sound.

Ton, or "sound," in the German language means both sound and matter.

- *Ton* means the clay that shapes the Earth.
- *Ton* means the sound that shapes our environment.

The book of Genesis says that God formed man from clay (or "dust"): "Streams came up from the earth and watered the whole surface of the ground. Then the Lord God formed a man of the dust of the ground and breathed into his nostrils the breath of life . . ." (NIV, Genesis 2:6–7).

The concept of **person** also leads us to the relationship between sound and human. Just like the previously explained concept of "resonance," which is also derived from Latin and stands for the "back-sounding" and "echoing." The original meanings of words indicate an aspect of life, according to which every being is also an echo, a vessel for vibrations, which it absorbs into itself, shapes, and swings back again into the world.

Person: Man (Latin, *persona,* "mask of the actor, role, represented by the mask"; *by,* "help to pass"; and *sonare,* "sound")

THE WORLD IN OUR EARS

The ear is our most **receptive** sense organ, keeping us in constant contact with our environment, our surroundings. Although the ear seems to be designed for the purpose of passively recording our impressions, it is like an antenna, always actively receptive to the world so as to fulfill its function. Perhaps evolution has made it so that we hear as soon as possible. This first sense of perception comes through waves and vibrations in the audible sound range of infrasound (below 16 herts) or ultrasound (above 16 kilohertz). In this sense, listening helps us survive.

> **Receptive:** Open and responsive to sensations, ideas, impressions; fit to receive and transmit stimuli

What we hear penetrates deep layers of the soul; therefore the ear is critical to information acquisition and processing. As early as 4.5 months after conception, the auditory organ in the growing fetus—the labyrinth and the cochlea—is already fully formed into its final size, proof that humans want to be able to hear as soon as possible. So before we are even an inch in length, still gestating in our mother's womb, we are already

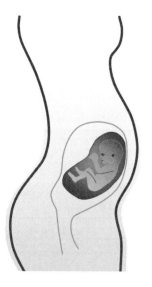

A person growing up in the shelter of the mother begins to hear.

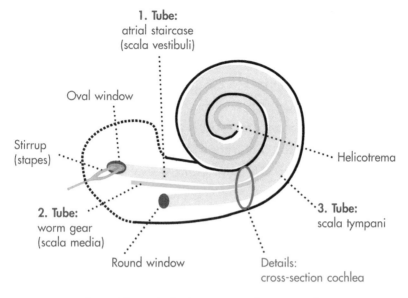

1. Tube:
atrial staircase
(scala vestibuli)

Oval window

Stirrup
(stapes)

Helicotrema

2. Tube:
worm gear
(scala media)

3. Tube:
scala tympani

Round window

Details:
cross-section cochlea

The cochlea, which also contains the organ of Corti

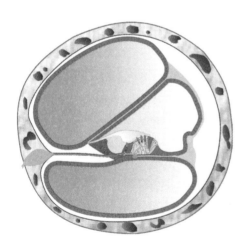

*Interior view (cross-section)
of the cochlea with its
3 tubes*

developing what will later become our two ears.[1] As mentioned before, this first physical development of our sense of hearing grows incredibly fast: 4.5 months later our actual hearing organ is already fully formed in its final size. In contrast, all the other features of the body continue to grow for many years after we are born, until around the age of 20. This proves that we want to hear ourselves in the womb, from the very beginning. Everything else we need for our development, our mother provides.

Our ability to hear while we're still in the womb affects our brain's development. Here's how: Anatomically, the organ of Corti, the receptor organ of hearing located in the cochlea, is the place where acoustic pulses are converted into electrical signals and then go through the neural pathways to the cerebral cortex.[2] On each of the approximately 20,000 sensory cells, the **Corti cells,** is a tuft of **cilia.** The cilia decode high-frequency sounds, thus supplying our brain with vital neural energy. Otolaryngologist Alfred A. Tomatis writes in his book:

> The first function of the ear is to ensure that the cortex receives sufficient neural energy through the "charging" effect of the ear. If a doctor overlooks this, it is because he is misguided by the generally accepted idea attributing an essentially auditory function to the ear. Indeed, this latter function is very much a secondary one. It is a well-known fact in zoology that the auditory apparatus acts as a charging or energizing dynamo. It furnishes current to feed the brain.[3]

Corti cells: The "hair cells," or receptors (sensory cells), of the inner ear, which convert stimuli into electrical activity. One differentiates the inner hair cells from the outer hair cells. Both are located in the organ of Corti, which forms an essential part of the cochlea.

Cilia: Also called *stereocilia*, these hair cells in the organ of Corti are up to 10 microns long and 0.25 micron wide (Latin, *cillum*, "eyelid, eyelashes"). They are the organelles that are responsible for hearing and balance.

The ear, through the **vestibule,** the inner ear labyrinth, provides 60 percent of these electrical charges, which enable us to regulate balance so that we can walk upright. The cochlea, the auditory cortex, adds another 30 percent of these stimuli, and together these structures charge the cerebral cortex.

Vestibule: The part of the inner ear that contributes principally to the sense of balance and spatial orientation for the purpose of coordinating movement with balance. Together with the cochlea, it constitutes the labyrinth of the inner ear (Latin, *vestibule*, "atrium, courtyard").

Through the ear we absorb vibrations, and sometimes we even listen between the lines and feel this unspoken vibration in our heart. If the words, the sounds, are soothing to us, beauty and the joy within us will be addressed. If the words are sharp and hurtful, we feel dissonance and pain. This also affects our balance and our sense of space. We then say, "That blew me away" or "I don't know which way is up and which way is down."

The vestibule is our main balance organ. Through the nerves of the spinal cord every muscle in the body communicates with the organ of balance, which unites with the nerve of the auditory organ. Thus the distribution of tension in the body, including muscle tone (cramping or laxity), posture, motor skills, and fine motor skills are regulated by the ear, which acts as a supervisory organ. One speaks of a cybernetic control loop consisting of the brain (issuing commands), the muscles (executing those commands), the ear (controlling the commands), and back again to the brain (correcting the commands as needed).

Thanks to our sense of hearing, we can fine tune and absorb information that allows us to empathize and resonate with what we hear around us. Aristotle described **mimesis** as the innate ability of humans to resonate. All sentient beings have the basic ability to empathize, to imitate, to mimic—to share experiences and re-create knowledge. This ability to resonate points to how we can self-regulate by learning how to move properly so as to restore hearing. The resonance within, the perception of what streams into and affects us, leads us to decide what is right for us when we learn how to listen to our inner self. The word mimesis also has another meaning as a physical gesture to achieve an effect. This points to the organization and effectiveness of our method, which requires a person to use proper movement to regulate the system of the body.

Mimesis: Mimicking, repeating the words or gestures of another (Greek, *mimeisthai,* "to imitate," and *mimos,* "mime")

HOW TRAUMA AFFECTS HEARING

Since the representative study of the German Tinnitus League [in] 1999, we know more details about the occurrence and impairment of tinnitus in Germany . . . at the time of investigation, nearly four million German citizens (over the age ten years) claimed to have been affected by tinnitus . . . According to a six-stage classification of severity, in Germany 1.5 million citizens suffered moderate to unbearable tinnitus.[4]

Tinnitus-Liga

According to the German Association of the Deaf, 14 million people are affected by hearing impairments.[5]

We don't just suddenly hear poorly for no apparent reason. The cause is always an event: we have experienced something that hurt us either physically or psychologically. What I hear can hurt quite a bit. Words can hurt us just like the loud *bang* of an explosion. If the injury that results from this kind of exposure does not heal completely, the functionality of the associated organ does not completely return to balance. Functionality is determined by two factors:

- **Quantity:** What quantity of hearing do I have left? For example, how many inner ear hairs are still able to process signals after an acoustic overload?
- **Quality:** To what extent can the organ concerned still do its job? What is the capacity of my entire system to develop a correct overall perception from less or incomplete information?

If we experience an event as **traumatic,** this affects the ear's physical functioning—I cannot make use of my system's full capabilities.

Similarly, the shock and pain of an acoustical traumatic event reduces my ability to process auditory information. In the past, the conventional medical model understood the causes of hearing impairment to be the result of inflammatory processes and diseases, genetic predisposition, or injury. It is certainly true that with old age there is often a weakening of the sense of hearing. An 80-year-old no longer hears exactly the same as a 15-year-old. But even given a significant weakening, it does not automatically mean that we cannot understand one another. There are usually reasons behind this other than the simplistic idea that our ears are worn out. And even with age-related deficits, old people, due to their experience and knowledge of life, can often compensate for a certain amount of hearing loss in a way that is not possible for a much younger person.

Traumatic, trauma: A wound, an injury, resulting in a disordered physical, psychic, or emotional state; exposure to violence, mental shock (Greek, *trauma*, "wound"). In psychology and psychiatry, trauma is the result of an externally acting violation of a person's psychic integrity.

If our body is injured, it can heal again as long as the affected organ is still present, nourished through the body's own supply channels, which are connected to the nervous system. This not only applies to our body as a whole but also, in a special way, to our sense of hearing. Our hearing system has enormous capabilities and is able to compensate for significant losses, meaning we have two ears that can perform independently of each other. If we experience a traumatic event, our entire body-mind-spirit reacts to it. The processing of the experience is similar to the input of certain commands on a computer keyboard. With an experience of this kind, one starts previously established and long-practiced chains of command in evolution. Such programs help us start to process traumatic events to ensure survival.

A traumatic event is always an overload to our system that leads to a weakening. However, what constitutes an overload is different for

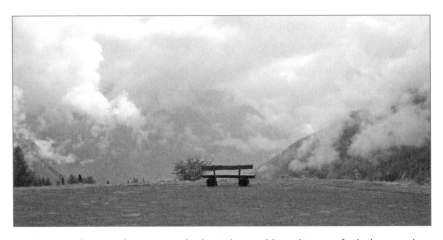

Trauma changes the way we look at the world, making us feel alone and isolated, such that the traumatic event itself is often clouded over and denied.

each person. For example, a heated argument with terrible insults may be deeply distressing for one person but may be insignificant to another. We might respond to verbal abuse with fear or anger, or we might shrug our shoulders and simply walk away. Depending on what we feel, the strain of the trauma is also felt differently in the body. However, if fear is the response to a trauma, an almost universal reaction is to freeze, to feel paralyzed. How strong this reaction is and how long it lasts depends on how deeply this fright has entered our psyche and "sits in our bones."

By understanding how we respond to trauma, we can make the processing and resolution of its physical **symptoms** more successful. The distinction between individual perception and universal processes is also crucial for scientific research to classify symptoms comprehensibly and to identify similar underlying causes with the same symptoms. This too is similar to a computer: it has a certain program that all users can access (and that program has a common structure), but what each individual calculates is very different.

Symptom: Subjective evidence of disease or physical or emotional disturbance (Greek, *symptoma,* "happening, attribute," from *syn* and *piptein,* "to fall").

THE 3 TYPES OF HEARING TRAUMA

The cause of hearing impairment involves any of 3 types of trauma:

- Accident, injury, or illness that results in a lasting impairment
- Physical overload of hearing as a result of a one-time (a loud explosion) or a sustained acoustic event (ongoing high level of noise in the workplace)
- A listening experience with traumatic emotional content (one-time or repeated verbal abuse)

Accident, Injury, Illness

Even if our hearing has been injured, it usually heals as long as the physical basics still exist, just as a cut on our finger heals eventually. Even if our hearing no longer functions perfectly as before, we still have the potential to restore it.

Let's consider a limited weakening of hearing; for example, in children after a middle-ear infection. The body may have healed from the illness, but on the soul level the shock of the illness has not yet been processed. So despite the fact that there has been a physical recovery, as a result of the shock to the system, the full functioning of auditory processing has not yet been restored. This is because restoration can only be done by the brain after it has processed the traumatic content on an emotional/soul/spirit level.

Hearing Loss Due to Blunt Trauma

A 47-year-old man told me this sad story: he had suffered a fractured skull at the age of 2 as a result of his father hitting him. Since then, he had been deaf in his left ear and suffered severe back and neck pain. This sturdy-looking man, a construction worker, looked like he could have been a boxer: he had a pulled-in, forward-tilted head, and his shoulders were angled forward in a protective stance, as if he always had to be careful not to be hit again.

Even after the first basic training session there was a significant change in his posture: his entire upper body was much more upright, and his neck pain was significantly reduced. The shift in the balance of his body had left him with a feeling of soreness in his upper body, especially his back, he said, as a result of the changes he was undergoing as his muscles started to adjust to the new posture. Even more significantly, his one-sided listening had changed, and he was now able to perceive sound on his supposedly deaf side. This was the beginning of him integrating his previously cut-off hearing side.

Physical Overload of Noise

In a physical overload of noise as a result of either a one-time stressful event or persistent stress (for example, high levels of noise in the workplace), the results are basically the same as with an accident or an injury.

Some years ago I presented my work on hearing regeneration to a gathering of friends and acquaintances. We had been sitting together for some time listening to music on my Naturschallwandler when one of the men who until then had been rather quiet spoke up: "There is a bit of bass missing," he said. I told him that our system doesn't work with the same kind of sound pressure the way conventional speakers do, resulting in a hearing sensation that is more intense, and I invited him to try it out. He then said that it would have little meaning for him because he had an accident many years ago, leaving him essentially deaf in his left ear. I asked him to sit down between the two speakers. Then I played the song "Over the Rainbow" by Eva Cassidy, so I could get an idea as to how his hearing field worked.

When I asked him where he heard the singer, he pointed to the right, just as I expected he would. I asked him if the volume was pleasant (as I had set the music a little louder than usual), and he said yes. I saw that he had relaxed and asked him after about a minute to align his head slightly forward as he continued to listen to the song. He suddenly asked, "Mr. Stucki, have you changed anything? The singer has moved." I said, "No, I did not change the music setting. What has changed is that your body geometry has started to work with the auditory information." I observed that his face was better supplied with blood, and he was alternatively visibly tense and then relaxed, which was a clear indication that his system typically interferes with audio information and was checking for the singer's location and beginning to adapt. Then I observed him looking to the right, and the singer was moved a bit more toward the center. At that moment he realized that he was experiencing sound from his left ear. He suddenly stood up and was so startled that he left the room.

Afterward his friend explained to me that during his training period in the army his comrades had fired a gun next to his left ear to scare him. He had suffered an acoustic trauma that had left him with a **perforation** of his eardrum, and since then he had heard nothing in that ear. Whether his inner ear was also damaged—which it very likely was—I did not know. Although at the time of the traumatic event all medical measures had been taken to restore his hearing in his left ear, it had not regulated again, and he'd been deaf in that ear ever since. Even if his eardrum had grown back,[6] it still didn't work as it did before. Also, the likely damage to the hair cells would have reduced his hearing. Yet the very fact that he was able to perceive the music coming from the area of his dramatic, unilateral hearing loss showed that a regeneration of the organ had taken place, or at the very least a residual function must have been preserved. However, since there had not been any improvement in his actual auditory perception on the injured side, it meant that the shock of many years past still "sits in his bones." He had not processed the long-ago event, the shock on both the mental and spiritual levels. Through our more-or-less chance encounter and the impact of the Naturschallwandler natural sound transducer, he was totally surprised and shocked to experience hearing on his left side.

> **Perforation:** A rather small rupture or tear. In most cases, the odds are very good that the tear will close up again by itself. Injuries with smooth wound edges usually heal well by themselves. If the tear has turned inside out, a doctor can smooth it

out and thus ensure a better wound healing. Whether surgical intervention is required depends on the size of the injury and the nature of the wound edges as well as the healing process. In about 85 percent of such cases no surgery is necessary. During the healing phase regular medical checkups are essential. If the injury is more than a quarter of the tympanic membrane surface, or if wound healing is taking longer than six weeks, surgery will be required. In a minor injury in which the wound edges are "rolled up," they are splinted by means of a silicone film. They can then grow back together more easily.

In the case of exposure to a sustained acoustic overload, exposure to the acoustic stressor must completely end so that the body can switch to regulation and regeneration mode. It's not important whether the acoustic burden is officially classified as harmful (for example, according to the requirements of occupational safety). The only decisive factor here is the subjective feeling of the listener. When a noisy environment or a certain type of noise (for example, the whirring and often high-frequency whistle emitted by certain ventilation and air-conditioning systems) is classified by one's own system as a burden or overload, then it *is* a threat to that person from a biological point of view, no matter what the actual decibel level is. The response of one's own body to the acoustic stressor is always based on individual sensation that is personally experienced. And it is only when we have discovered and solved the traumatic background that we can begin to deal with the stress brought on by that trauma. Processing the causes of trauma will be discussed throughout this book.

So the individual's personal response to acoustic stress is paramount. And it usually is not enough to reduce the exposure to stressful noise with hearing protection because the noise is subjectively still perceived as a burden, even when the sound is objectively lower due to the protective measures. Let's consider a worker with an angle grinder. By working without adequate hearing protection, his hearing has been reduced. He recognizes this and always wears ear protection, which objectively reduces the level of noise. However, at this point the stress is no longer linked to the volume of the noise. In other words, it doesn't matter if the lion is far away and therefore can only be heard softly or if he's close and therefore sounds louder; in both cases there is a potential hazard based on how the body reacts.

Therefore, first and foremost, the external noise load must be completely eliminated. This is often difficult in practice when it comes to a noisy job or a living situation where one is continuously exposed to noise (such as living near a road or an airport). Often people think that if the noise is considered below what's considered allowable stress levels, they feel they should just accept the burdensome situation; that's because they don't understand the subjective factor in hearing trauma.

Also note how phrases like "Don't be so sensitive!" "What do you want?" and "We have done everything" might be well-intentioned but don't help recognize the true issue of the situation. They're often only a further burden and generally only lead to weakened self-worth and self-esteem of the affected people.

Of course you can also work in parallel with some form of therapy while you reconstruct your sense of hearing, but if you are still exposed to the overload of noise, the therapy is usually not particularly effective because your perceptual system will continue to view the acoustic stress as a burden and remain in protective mode.

On the other hand, someone who works without hearing protection and regularly uses a tool like an angle grinder or a circular saw might find that their brain reduces the burden of the subjective perception of noise, such that the noise is no longer heard as loud or disruptive. As a child, I used to live on a street with a tram. Very often, when it went around the bend, it squeaked. At first, I woke up startled. After a few weeks, though, I barely registered the squeaky sound when the tram went by. I had gotten used to the sound, my system recognized it as familiar and nonthreatening, and so my system had hidden the high-pitched frequencies so that they wouldn't bother me anymore. This is also how it might work if you regularly use a power tool.

However, if you stop using the angle grinder regularly, you'd have to teach your brain to hear those frequencies again, since your system has learned to block out those frequencies. This kind of retraining often feels strange in the beginning because your whole system is focused on *not* hearing those frequencies, and so it doesn't. This is what allowed you to handle the situation in the past. In addition, if those frequencies have been especially loud and burdensome, your system might have been weakened within this range of frequency on a physical and organic level.

A Hunter with Hearing Loss

An outdoorsman in his early 70s who had hunted all his life could no longer hear notes in the high frequency as a result of the damage resulting from shotgun noise, such that when he went into the forest he couldn't hear the sounds of the birds and other critters any longer. This pained him greatly.

We trained intensively, using the basic method described in chapter 5. During this time he discontinued the sport of hunting. At the end of the training I played him a special CD with different bird sounds, and after a while I observed tears running down his cheeks. He had been told by doctors that he must accept the fact that he would never again hear the sound of the birds, and yet now he heard their melodies.

I told him that were he to resume shooting for sport, his hearing problem would most likely return and he would not be able to hear the birds again. We discussed this in detail—he had to decide right then and there whether he was going to change his life—whether his love of shooting was greater than his love of hearing the birds and other sounds of the forest. He opened up and told me that he had increasingly been having difficulty shooting—"not because of the loud bang, but to see the death that comes from my hand—it bothers me."

In this case, it was not so easy to just say, "I have a problem with shooting, but I want both to be able to shoot and to hear the birds." The man could not have both. He also had to ask himself whether hunting animals was still right for him.

Sometime later, he called me and said he was very happy hearing the birds in the forest. When I asked, "And what about shooting?" He replied, "Shooting? Yes, I now have a great camera, and I shoot photos of the birds as often as I can."

To hear is indeed to listen: What does the world want to tell me? I have to listen to that too. What does my inner voice say? Do I have to change anything? As a good friend of mine said, "The nice thing about attitudes is that you can adjust them."

Listening Experience with Traumatic Emotional Content

Traumatic events do not necessarily involve physical force. Our soul and consciousness are involved in every event. How our soul perceives an event is of utmost importance and determines our consciousness. In conjunction with the brain, the soul and consciousness process sensory impressions absorbed by the body. If your internal perceptions don't agree with your external reality, you may not be able to accurately locate or perhaps even hear certain frequencies. This kind of listening trauma, which is often indistinguishable from trauma resulting from organic impairments or accidents, can be caused by emotionally traumatic acoustic events.

With the basic training method we have developed an approach for the treatment of hearing disorders that goes beyond a purely organic diagnosis and follows a more holistic approach. The physical component is not the only deciding factor, and not every painful situation affects a person physically. We'll deal with that in the next section.

IT HITS ME: WHERE DO I NOTICE IT IN THE BODY?

Three Ways an Experience Manifests in the Body

Life entails experiencing conflict from time to time. Arguing with our partner, getting angry at work, becoming resentful when someone insults us or unfairly accuses us—an emotional upset might make us feel that *I don't think I'm hearing this right!* or *I can't believe my ears!* These are the kinds of feelings we may have when we experience conflicts connected to our auditory system. Sometimes such situations have a physical component; more often they don't. Not every conflict strikes us in the pit of our stomach, but sometimes a physical reaction is an indicator that something just doesn't sit right with us and even overwhelms us.

A listening experience involving emotional trauma brings three factors together in a single moment:

- shock (surprised),
- isolation (one feels alone at the moment), and
- acute and dramatic personal threat (the situation has significance for us at the moment).

If these factors occur in an accident or injury, the natural healing process is hampered, or at least very slow. Before I explain the three factors in more detail, I'll first give you another example of an emotionally traumatic and biologically active situation of our practice.

Childhood Tinnitus as a Result of Father's Criticism

Wolfgang, a man in his 40s, told me that he can still remember how his tinnitus started. When he was 6 years old the family went on a skiing holiday. His father had always had high expectations for him and impressed these upon him: Wolfgang had to be among the best and learn everything as well as his father. Above all, he should not be a coward.

Wolfgang recalled having to take the ski lift one morning after a short period of "practice" that consisted mostly of his father saying, "You'll learn, it's easy!"

"As we stood in line and I saw how far the chair lift went up the mountain, I got scared," he said. "I didn't want to go up there,

and I told my father so. Then he snapped, yelling at me in front of everyone: 'You weakling, you sissy!' My mother, who was standing a little farther back in the line, didn't do anything to help me. I couldn't move for I don't know how long—all I knew was that suddenly there was a sound in my ear."

Unless accidents or injuries have occurred, diseases and the dramatic weakening of our systems and capabilities always start with situations or events that were too much for us. These catch us off guard, or are the final straw, so to speak. When we have to deal with all three factors (shock, isolation, and acute and dramatic personal threat) within a single cognitive event at once, that experience becomes existential and kickstarts our body's survival program—our last resort, one could say.

- **Shock:** A shock can result in a state of paralysis—I freeze. The situation is so powerful that I have no idea what I can do or how I can escape it or resolve it. It's like the mouse that turns the corner and unexpectedly faces the cat. It instinctively senses that any movement could mean death. If it moves, the cat will be on it, so the mouse freezes. Like the poor mouse, the event catches us completely off guard—it's something we didn't expect at all.

- **Isolation:** This is the feeling of being all alone in the world, without any help or support, no matter how many people may be around. If the little fawn is separated from its mother, it is isolated, which poses the highest level of risk. If the mother can't find the fawn it is without any support for survival. Isolation from the group or family can mean mortal danger. If my boss puts me down in front of the whole team, I will feel isolated from my colleagues, and this will make me feel that my very survival at work is threatened.

- **Personal threat:** This means that the situation or the event has some meaning to me personally. It's about something important to me. As a result, I lose face, I feel that I'm worthless, that I'm no longer loved, that I've lost everything. The situation represents a threat, so I cannot just ignore it.

When the triggering event combines feelings of shock, isolation, and high drama, our entire system becomes overloaded. When these three factors come together in a situation where what we hear is part of the conflict, an essential aspect of the whole event, our sense of hearing can become impaired. In other words, our sense of hearing can become seriously weakened if we have experienced one or more situations in which these three factors came together and restricted our sense of hearing. A constant drip of water wears away the stone.

We can heal this kind of trauma by processing the triggering event, which helps to strengthen our sense of hearing. I'm not saying that it's easy, but it's worth it, and in each of us there is more strength and resilience than we sometimes think. A central aspect for me to mobilize this force is in understanding the contexts so that I can gain confidence that this work makes sense because it is in accordance with the order of nature.

DISORDERS OF THE EAR
Diverse and Yet Connected

To review, the complex process of hearing is connected to symmetry and balance. Symmetry is an essential basis for the proper functioning of our body. Asymmetry—the displacement of the body axes—generally weakens our hearing and is an expression of how unevenly we hear on both sides. With an unbalanced posture it is much more difficult to build a complete—that is, symmetrical—sense of hearing.

Symmetry and balance control our bodily movements via the corresponding organ in the inner ear, the vestibule. This organ of equilibrium is also directly involved in spatial location because we must always know our own orientation in space—whether we are lying down or standing, whether and how much our head is tilted—to correctly relate to sounds in space. Symmetry and balance are associated with the reference point at the back of the head, from which we build our listening field. A weakening of our hearing is always associated with symmetry and balance.

Let us now consider 3 special cases of hearing disorders.

Tinnitus: Have I done something wrong?

Tinnitus, the subjective sensation of a noise such as a high-pitched ring-ing, hum, knocking, or a roaring that can only be heard by the one affected, has become a widespread problem.[7]

The reasons for the increase in this condition have not been clearly established by conventional medicine. There are, of course, environmen-tal and physiological causes such as loud noise or inflammation of the ear. Holistic medicine has found that a trigger for tinnitus can also be a traumatic life event. Last but not least, stress is considered a signifi-cant factor; however, in our work with hearing we have found that stress is not exactly a trigger but more a booster of the existing noise of the tinnitus.

Our approach to understanding the causes of tinnitus assumes that there is an acoustic signal created by the brain due to a traumatic experi-ence. The assumption that tinnitus actually occurs in the brain is sup-ported by cases in which the perceived sound in the ear could not be stopped, even by cutting or severing the auditory nerve. This aside, it is always important to fix any purely physical causes such as tension, espe-cially in the neck and shoulders, if it is found to be a factor in the tinnitus.

In addition to the enormous burden of never-ending noise in the ear, those who are affected by this condition often have difficulty cor-rectly orienting themselves to their environment. They no longer accu-rately perceive where a sound is coming from and how they themselves are involved in an acoustic event. A subtle sense of insecurity and even threat arises as a result, along with social isolation that comes from not being involved in the surrounding environment. Even if you have learned to live with the noise, there is often a fear that the tinnitus could grow worse, to the point where you can no longer cope.

At its core I consider tinnitus to be an event that represents the physical manifestation of a mental conflict. Therefore, the best approach is to resolve the underlying theme to establish new regulation and heal-ing. This is true in the following case, in which there is ostensibly an organic cause of the tinnitus.

Eardrum Burst during a Concert

Mr. S.: *"At a concert my eardrum burst and since then I have tinnitus."*

We all notice when something is not good for us, when we go beyond our limits, be it physical limits or the limits of social pressure ("Come on, don't act like that!"). Such was the case of Mr. S., who, against his better judgment attended a loud rock concert, whereupon his eardrum burst. It's not uncommon in such a situation for self-condemnation to arise: "If I hadn't gone to that concert, I wouldn't have suffered that injury. That was a big mistake."

Of course, conventional medicine declared that the eardrum had burst because it was too loud at the concert. But why didn't the eardrum heal? Why did it turn into the never-ending noise of tinnitus? If the cause was only mechanical, everyone at the concert would have had the same injury to the ears; however, this was clearly not the case. So the crucial issue was not a physical overload due to the volume of the music but rather Mr. S.'s self-condemnation and unprocessed shock.

We all make mistakes. It's part of life. It is important that we do not give up or resign ourselves to being at fault but begin to process the error. Tinnitus is like a wound that doesn't heal because the thoughts and fears that are associated with the triggering event have not been resolved.

We have found that working on healing tinnitus—especially when you've been suffering from strong ear noises for a long time and hear the ringing constantly—requires a lot of patience. We usually speak of a period of 1 to 2 years before we can get relief. The reason is because such a long-lasting condition always reflects conflicts in key areas of life. Resolving these life issues takes time, knowledge, and implementation in real life. It's hard work that takes a lot of energy, but such therapeutic work also provides opportunities and a new vision of the meaning and goals of one's life.

The subject of tinnitus would no doubt provide material for a whole separate book. It involves working in progressive steps, which I will sketch below to provide an overview of what's involved. Of course, there's always the possibility that this condition will simply disappear; however, it's best not to create these kinds of expectations, because the hope for instantaneous relief generates pressure and counteracts the process of healing.

Basically, tinnitus is the result of a conflict of self-worth, of how you feel about yourself: *Am I correct? Can I do it? I can't solve this!*

Daughter Refuses to See Mother in Hospital

Mrs. G. told me about the start of her tinnitus: "Some years ago I was in the hospital. Ever since then I've had tinnitus. So far I've always thought that the cause was incorrectly administered medication. By thinking back as to whether the cause could be psychological, I immediately remembered something. While in the hospital I asked my good friend and neighbor to inform my daughter, with whom I had no contact for 15 years. When my friend came back to the hospital to see me the next day she told me that my daughter had asked her, 'Is it life-threatening?' My friend told her that it was serious but not life-threatening. Then my daughter said, 'Then I'm not coming.' That hit me really hard. Shortly after that, the tinnitus started."

The following steps for the relief of the tinnitus phenomenon may serve as a guide to gaining insight and eventual healing:

1. *What do I want?* What state do I want to achieve? This doesn't mean explaining what you don't want but rather defining where you do wish to go, what you want out of life in general.

2. *Inventory the noise:* What sounds do I hear exactly (a knocking, a whistling)? On which side of my head do I perceive the noise?

3. *History and chronology:* Since when have I heard the noise? When did the noise occur for the first time? When did the sound change? Are there situations, times of the day, when the sound changes? Did new sounds come along?

4. *Time of inception:* What was the situation when the noise first came about? How did I feel? What happened? The idea here is to explore the triggering event for the tinnitus and to find out what happened. What feelings and thoughts did I have at the

time? Often there are thoughts and feelings of guilt and failure.

5. *Establishment of a listening area:* After following steps 1 through 4, we now have a starting point. Chapter 5 is a complete review of the basic therapeutic method, including the training of spatial orientation and the full establishment of the listening field. Often an improvement in tinnitus occurs by this act of self-regulation. It may be that an intact hearing field already exists or adjusts itself without the noise significantly changing. However, a correct listening field is always a prerequisite for further work.

6. *Body geometry:* This involves the resolution of physical causes such as tension. If, for example, certain head positions intensify the tinnitus, these physical tensions must be worked on. This book includes various exercises; as well, the expert hands of a professional **osteopath, chiropractor,** or sensitive healer can sometimes work wonders.

Osteopath: A person who practices osteopathy, a system of medical practice based on the theory that diseases are due chiefly to loss of structural integrity, which can be restored by manipulation of the parts, supplemented by other therapeutic measures (Greek, *osteon,* "bone," and *pathos,* "suffer")

Chiropractor: A licensed health care professional who treats disorders of the musculoskeletal system (such as back and neck pain) usually through the manual adjustment or manipulation of the spinal vertebrae to correct nervous system dysfunction (Greek, *khavr,* "hand")

7. *Identify and document changes:* When is the tinnitus stronger? When does it weaken? Of particularly importance is observing which situations and events put me in stress and therefore strengthen the tinnitus. For this you should keep a diary with

exact times and dates, in which all changes in both the intensity and the nature of the sound are recorded.

8. *Identify conflict issues:* Find out exactly when the tinnitus started and what the exact conflict-related issue is. Tinnitus is caused by an emotional trauma that was overwhelming and unsolvable at the moment and since then is more or less latent. The conflict is like a record that has gotten scratched and now always repeats the same theme. If the conflict is not resolved, the regeneration of hearing can take place only on the physical plane, as with the healing of eardrum scarring, but the emotional underpinnings will remain; so without addressing the inner, deep-seated conflict the noise will remain.

9. *Resolve the conflict and therefore the tinnitus:* For details on how to do this, see chapter 6 (pages 200 through 204).

10. *New life, new ways:* You can do this all by yourself . . .

Vertigo: This Will Blow Me Over

The underlying emotional source of dizziness is usually a very stressful and prolonged life situation that I want to back out of—at the same time, I think that I may not be able to. I'm in a kind of **dilemma** that involves a permanent state of tension. Again, as always, try to exclude purely physical causes; for example, a shift of the crystals in the semicircular canals in what is known as vestibular vertigo, the so-called positional vertigo.

> **Dilemma:** A predicament (such as between two evils), a difficulty (Greek, *dilemma*, "double bind")

The basic therapeutic method that I present in detail in chapter 5 has proved to be a very helpful way to work with dizziness to reduce its effects in our daily lives. This is partly because I've learned in this training to accurately and consciously perceive and control my body. Dizziness is always a loss of fine motor control of the body's system that regulates balance and movement. In standing and walking, our body is in a constant dynamic regulation process; it always fluctuates around a center, and to maintain balance it's constantly fine-tuning various balancing movements. Again, these muscle regulations aim to accurately perceive movements and to move with much less effort.

The following breathing exercise is not related to any particular breathing technique. It involves breathing normally and observing how your body acts during inhalation and exhalation.

EXERCISE: Breathing Consciously

Simply follow your natural breathing rhythm, without manipulating the breath.

Thoughts may come, and if so, allow them to pass and return to the task of observing your breath. Do this exercise with your eyes open or closed, however you are most comfortable, for 3 minutes. To keep track of time try using a small hourglass, which is not as abrupt as the ringing of a timer. Observe how your body feels after the exercise.

Comments and hints: Commit your undivided attention to perceiving and observing your breath and not being distracted by thoughts, which is difficult for most people. This is a basic meditation exercise. We recommend that you do this exercise over a period of 21 days or longer, and try doing it once or twice a day, to see how it affects your life. If you like it, you will then find your own rhythm.

As we know, the ability to detect whether a sound source moves—for example, whether the engine noise comes from a moving or a stationary car, or whether the singer I'm listening to moves in the room or not—is an important part of our sense of hearing. This skill is part of our survival equipment. If a noise source is not moving but I perceive it as moving, then this might trigger or reinforce my dizziness. Bringing the correct location of the noise source back into line with what we hear is an important aspect of the regulation of vertigo.

Depending on the strength of dizziness issue we have to be very careful and must go slowly. It's all about long-term stabilization and not short-term success. If the exercises and training while standing are too difficult, then we start while sitting. If it still feels very unsafe when we close our eyes, then we start with open eyes. If the practice seems too strenuous to do for several minutes, we start with a shorter time. What's important here, as with all the other exercises, is that we create a sense of security so that we can process gradually according to our own needs.

Hyperacusis: Acute Sensitivity to Sound

People who suffer from the symptoms of hyperacusis, an acute sensitivity to sound, especially certain sounds, have at some point in some way been frightened to death. They perceived a threat that overwhelmed them and decided not to hear it. With hyperacusis, you actually hear things that others can't or do not perceive as a noise burden. This hypersensitivity is no improvement in hearing in the sense of strengthening, however, because it is an overstimulation of auditory perception, similar to having very sensitive skin and wearing a garment that constantly irritates the skin. This overstimulation is often perceived as very painful and can lead to severe hearing loss. These people are in a constant state of tension to avoid being surprised by loud noises, or they withdraw into a space as quiet as possible because the usual noise of everyday life is too painful for them to bear. They seek a "cave" in which to find security through seclusion from the world.

When considering the symptoms we must try to figure out what they're telling us. It's basically this: *I don't miss any noise. I hear the smallest of sounds, so nothing can surprise, threaten, or overwhelm me. I can now avoid the worst that has happened to me and I no longer have to experience it.* People with hyperacusis are often sensitive beings who have experienced bad things in early childhood. Building trust and a cautious approach is necessary for them, especially if they have experienced this level of hypersensitivity for several years and are therefore highly defensive.

The Clattering Sounds of the Kitchen

Mr. L. is a young man in his early 20s with strong hyperacusis. The clattering sounds of dishes, kitchen utensils, and pots and pans are especially disturbing to him. When we first met, his sensitivity had already reached a level that made it painful for him to eat with other people. The food sounds, especially the quiet scraping and clattering of spoons, cups, and forks, were so unbearable to him that his system reacted with a strong temporary hearing loss, while at the same time he fell into a sort of rigidity in which he could only move in slow motion. His movements froze as if someone had flipped a switch. After many conversations, including some that involved his mother, we explored what the causes of his hypersensitivity might be. The following picture emerged.

In his first 2 years of his life his mother always kept him in a small cot in the kitchen while she was busy cooking. His father was a violent man, and his older brother often came into the kitchen, where some very ugly scenes ensued, with shouting and physical violence, dishes smashed, and so forth. Finally his mother left the home and took the young Mr. L. with her to live in a women's shelter until she could find a permanent living situation. In recounting this period of time the mother said that her young son had fewer and fewer movements, which she didn't notice until someone pointed out that he was virtually motionless and had become very thin as well.

In the women's shelter and afterward, the young Mr. L. was always a bit quieter than other boys his age. He was sensitive to sound, but without showing any other abnormalities. That changed later in life when he began an apprenticeship as a cook, which he completed successfully, after which he continued to work in a big kitchen. There he had a male and a female boss, both of whom constantly argued about the right strategy and who had what skills and what to do. With this new situation he gradually became more and more sensitive to the sounds of the kitchen, until he couldn't stand it anymore and finally had to leave the job.

Healing hyperacusis is a gradual process that takes time, patience, and perseverance. If possible it's always helpful if both parents can be involved if the hyperacusis is connected with them.

With any disorder of the ear, to address the issue of what made me so painfully sensitive is all the more possible, the more I deal with the general context of the development of physical pathologies. As a result, a knowledge arises that there can be a resolution of the pain!

4

Everything
Has a Beginning

The History of Sound Research

ALL WE CAN DO WE ONCE LEARNED

Everything we have learned in our lifetime we have learned consciously. Even as a baby we were essentially a great mind in a small body; we wanted to explore the world around us. In the beginning, we didn't know how to move and control our body, so everything was quite awkward. Listening, feeling, touching, being touched—that was our world as a newborn. So many new things. As a toddler we quickly learned: turn around, sit, crawl. We pulled ourselves up using a chair leg while our proud mom and dad proclaimed, "Oh look, she's standing!" It wasn't long before we took our first steps.

All this developed out of our inner drive to move, to run. What a feeling! This impulse didn't happen with the conscious thought, *I will now learn to walk,* yet it was a conscious process, albeit one not tied to words. The desire to expand our space, to see the world, was our driving force.

Do you remember your first steps as a child? Do you remember how proud you were? Every person knew intuitively how to accomplish these first steps. It started with small movements: *grab my foot, take my toes in*

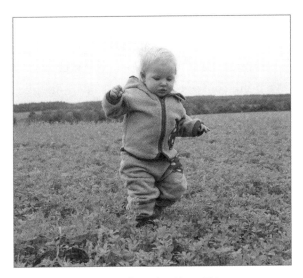

First steps. Photo by Mara Ebinger.

my mouth, feel that the foot belongs to me, see what happens . . . To learn we had to initiate this process of repetition, correction, and many other movement sequences that eventually led to our first steps.

All learning takes place in steps. Learning is being conscious of being able to change something or do something that I may not have been able to do or know before. This is true for restoring one's hearing. If I hear badly now, I probably have the habit of thinking, *I hear badly.* Because this is my experience, I "know" it, and I experience it that way. That's a problem, however. What I do not "know" is that bad hearing (or bad listening) has its reason. We once learned to hear, and then we forgot how to. Once we learn to ride a bike, there would have to be an underlying reason why we couldn't ride one later. Most hearing deficits are like that.

We have already seen how the source of hearing deficits usually lies somewhere in the past, perhaps in a single event, perhaps in many small events. Sometimes people who hear badly are actually thinking, *I don't want to hear anything anymore.* Why do they not want to hear anything? Is it really so, or do they think that only to avoid feeling all the pain and loss?

All that we can do we once had to learn. If I want to change a weakness or an undesirable condition, it is necessary to go to the point where it began to understand the reasons why it exists and what I can do about it. We don't consciously unlearn something like hearing, but if something hurts, we fight it off. That's a perfectly natural reaction. This repulsion and suppression of pain is a decision, otherwise we would not be able to reverse it—and we *can* reverse it. To regenerate our hearing, it is important that we realize *why* our hearing can improve. Understanding is an important building block. It's not about a great method by which people suddenly hear again. It's about the process of knowledge: "Everything is in me. Yes, I basically created this myself, and if I'm aware of the origin of the hearing loss, the pain, the defensiveness, and the repression, then functionality can come back. Then I can heal—then I can heal *myself*, as I have done many times before."

If I don't understand why hearing can be improved, then I can't believe it can be. Then it is a coincidence whether hearing improves. To recognize what has been learned by scientists over time, that there is a natural order, is part of the foundation to understanding that hearing regeneration is not a coincidence. Join me on a short trip through history in this chapter, knowing that if I can understand why, then I can believe, and I can therefore change my situation. This doesn't mean that it's easy, but there is definitely a possibility that *I can do it!*

WHAT WE ARE TODAY HAS BEEN GOING ON FOR THOUSANDS OF YEARS

If you want to understand the secrets of the universe, think in terms of energy, frequency and vibration.

Nikola Tesla

The earliest peoples, our ancient ancestors, created sounds and made music. Music, singing, and sounds have always been expressed by all cultures in a spiritual context. Sounds and vibrations were associated with the possibility of connecting with a higher self, as in a voice raised in prayer or ritual music and song.

Over time, people recognized that sounds were also associated with the geometry of certain ways of building. In ancient Greece, master builders succeeded in achieving a sound distribution in their amphitheaters via special architecture that allowed an audience of several thousand people, without any amplification technology, to clearly hear and understand a performer from every seat in the theater so that many people were included in a common experience. This achievement was realized through the correct observation and implementation of natural phenomena in connection with spiritual knowledge of sacred geometry and sound. A perfect example is the theater of Epidaurus, which dates back to the 4th century BCE.

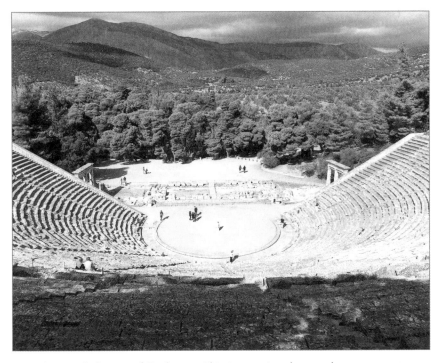

The amphitheater of Epidaurus. This impressive theater that seats up to 14,000 people is built on a slope and is still the most prominent building in the ancient Greek city of Epidaurus. It has excellent acoustics, such that even in the back rows people can clearly understand every word spoken on stage. Photo by Christian Glück.

Our research into how to restore hearing naturally actually goes back thousands of years. We have always felt that sound touches deep layers in sentient beings and that matter communicates through vibrations. If I knock on wood, the sound is very different from when I hammer on stone. Each being and each element has its own language, its own vibration. This is particularly illustrated by the following example from the animal world: In South Georgia, a group of islands located east of the southern tip of South America, 200,000 to 400,000 king penguins breed every year when the adult penguins come back from fishing for food for themselves and their young. Upon their return from the sea they need to find their young among the thousands of young penguins, all looking completely alike. They find them only by hearing. They call their babies from afar, and the young penguins respond with their own unique cheeping cries.

Pythagoras

Some of our knowledge of sound was built on our knowledge of numbers. More than 2,500 years ago, the Greek philosopher Pythagoras recognized that the starry sky reproduces musical harmonies and integer numbers. Each of the seven known (at that time) planets was assigned a single tone of the seven-note scale. Pythagoras found through experiments on a **monochord** that there is a clear relationship between numbers and sounds.

Monochord: An ancient Greek musical instrument with a single string over a resonant body and a scale in which points along the string are delineated to give certain notes (Greek, *monochordon*, from *monos*, "alone"; and *chorda*, "string")

Dividing the string of the monochord right in the middle—that is, the ratio of 1 to 2—the new tone is now an octave higher but sounds quite similar to the base note. The individual sounds of our Western scale have been created by dividing a particular string length into 12

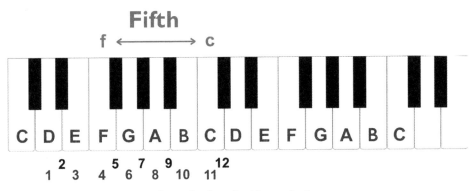

Piano keyboard with numbering

equal sections. This can be seen very clearly on a piano keyboard. The 7 white keys and 5 black keys make a total of 12, or one complete octave. The next octave begins in the same pattern. Through this orderly structure, all individual keys are in a specific mathematical relationship with one another. Pythagoras's theory is based on the idea that all things are based on numbers and numerical relationships. From this followed the realization that music is not determined by the individual sounds but rather on the relationship between the sounds and the circumstances. Notably, every child in ancient Greece was educated in a way that we can barely imagine today. By the age of 11 at the latest, a child would have mastered 2 to 3 instruments, as recorded by Greek historian Herodotus (484–425 BCE).

The connection between sound and its form of expression, vibration, inevitably led to the perception of an order that permeates and acts on everything. We intuitively perceive and feel this order and therefore are part of this order. We're not lost in a chaotic and incomprehensible universe. We exist within this order, which is expressed through vibration and always reveals new layers—just as sound that builds up through the formation of more and more overtones.

Johannes Kepler

German astronomer, mathematician, and astrologer Johannes Kepler (1571–1630) observed that the planetary gears in our solar system correspond to **harmonic** intervals. The idea of order eventually led him, through meticulous observation, to three basic laws concerning gravity, space, and time, on which we still calculate our calendar and the movements of the sun and the moon. Is it not a small wonder that we can predict the next full moon with utmost precision, that we know when the longest day is, and even know when the next time the moon moves in front of the sun in a solar eclipse, bringing darkness to the Earth during daytime?

Harmonic: Following the fixed laws of harmony; a component frequency of a complex wave that is an integral multiple of the fundamental frequency (Greek, *harmonia*, "harmony")

Kepler discovered a fundamental law of nature, that all planets move in ellipses, with the sun as a focus—Kepler's first law of planetary motion. Kepler's second law of planetary motion relates to the

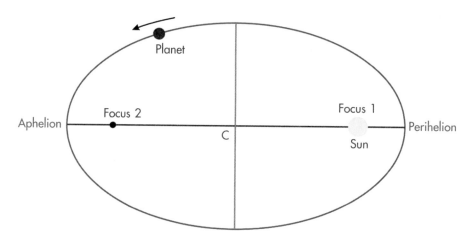

Perihelion: point of the orbit in which   C = center of the ellipse
a planet is closest to the sun
Aphelion: point of the orbit in which
a planet is farthest from the sun

Kepler understood that the solar system corresponds to harmonic intervals. Kepler's first law of planetary motion states that planets move in an elliptical orbit around the sun. Kepler's laws show the relationships that occur when everything moves around and is defined by 1 point. From this, order builds.

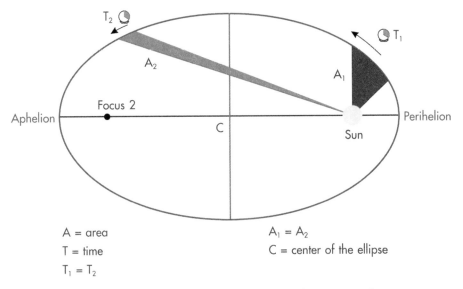

A = area
T = time
$T_1 = T_2$

$A_1 = A_2$
C = center of the ellipse

Kepler's second law of planetary motion states that space and time are in a fixed relationship. When objects move, there's always a universal order in their relationship.

connection between area and time. It shows that every planet orbiting the sun always defines an equal area (sector) in the same period of the ellipse, regardless of which part of its orbit around the sun it occupies—in other words, planets sweep out equal areas in equal times. His third law of planetary motion reaches further into the order of the universe, revealing even deeper layers: the square of the orbital period of a planet is directly proportional to the cube of the semimajor axis of its orbit—a law that captures the relationship between the distance of planets from the sun and their orbital periods. In these laws Kepler recognized the relationship between space and time. All three laws apply to all possible combinations of planets in our solar system.[1]

As applied to our work, Kepler's laws show the relationship and the interaction of 1 point (everything moves around 1 point and is defined by this), from which an order builds. When a second moving point is added, there's always a universal order in the structure of their relationship. However different this relationship might be, how far these points are from each other, how long the points need to move around

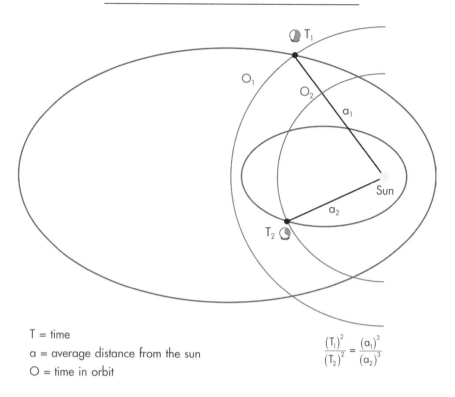

T = time

a = average distance from the sun

O = time in orbit

$$\frac{(T_1)^2}{(T_2)^2} = \frac{(a_1)^3}{(a_2)^3}$$

Kepler's third law of planetary motion captures the relationship between the distance of planets from the sun and their orbital periods. The further a planet from the sun, the longer that planet takes to orbit the sun. All relationships in the universe are precise.

each other, all these relationships follow a common order in time and motion. Building on this concept, the order of space and time now follows irrefutably. Or more simply: if we have a reference point, it is easier to find and define a point outside of ourselves, which then results in a new and clear orientation in space. In short, time and distance are linked. The longer a stretched string, the slower it vibrates when it is set in motion. The shorter the string, the faster it vibrates and the higher its sound is to our ears.

Ernst Chladni

German physicist and musician Ernst Chladni (1756–1827) invented a technique that made the relationship between sound and vibration

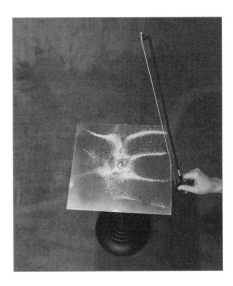

A bow is pulled against a plate, causing it to vibrate into resonance and create a pattern.

visible. His technique consisted of drawing a bow over a piece of metal whose surface was lightly covered with sand. Vibration caused the sand to move and concentrate along the lines where the surface was still. The patterns formed by these lines are what are now called Chladni figures.

In his groundbreaking 1787 work, *Entdeckungen über die theorie des klanges* [Discoveries in the theory of sound], Chladni described vibrations and stressed that sound and sound theory should not be treated as a study of air, as had previously happened, but instead that it should be considered in terms of the periodic oscillations of elastic bodies.

Hans Jenny

Swiss naturalist Hans Jenny (1904–1972) took Chladni's discoveries further, coining the term **cymatics** to describe the acoustic effects of sound-wave phenomena. Jenny experimented with technically produced oscillation patterns: specifically, the surface of a plate, diaphragm, or membrane is vibrated, and regions of maximum and minimum displacement are made visible in a thin coating of particles, paste, or liquid. Different patterns emerge depending on the geometry of the plate and the driving frequency. His repeatable experiments allowed him to systematically investigate vibration and matter. His images of flowing media were

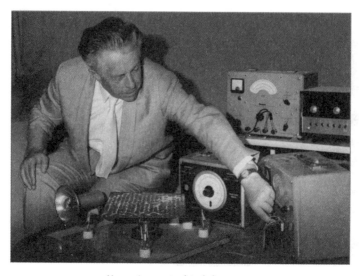

Hans Jenny in his laboratory.
Photo from the book Kymatik *by Hans Jenny*
(AT Verlag: Baden, 2009).

sonicated tones reminiscent of forms that are familiar to us from nature. Not only do regular and round figures emerge, but patterns also periodically repeat in one direction and resemble the blueprint of a skeleton.

Cymatics: The study of sound and vibration made visible, typically on the surface of a plate, diaphragm, or membrane (Greek, *kyma*, "wave")

In 1967, Jenny published the first volume of his work *Kymatic,* and in 1972 he published the second volume. These works show in an impressive way how vibrations generate forms and interact with one another. Both volumes of *Kymatic* are foundational for understanding resonance and when and how vibrations act and shape matter.

Notably, if the vibrating membrane is no longer moved the same way, and the frequencies and the strength (amplitude) are varied, more complex wormlike bodies appear to glide across the plate. This is a demonstration of how ancient myths describe the conception of our physical world taking shape through sound.

Theodor Schwenk

Jenny's contemporary, engineer and anthroposophist Theodor Schwenk (1910–1986), a noted water researcher, devoted himself to the study of the interaction between fluids and the pathogenesis of forms as a result of mutual penetration. Where a body is, there cannot be another. However, the most diverse movements can penetrate the same location, as already shown. Thus only one body can exist in any one place, but many, even multidimensional, movements may be present.

Examples of shape formation are found in a liquid that is penetrated by a second liquid. We may think of these fluids as vibrations or as impulses that interact with each other and work together to create an order. A stream that flows briskly over stones forms countless inner surfaces and vortices. By absorbing moving water from the earth and from plants, animals, and humans, the water passes on these received impressions and communicates them in subtle patterns. Thus with Schwenk's work we come to a finer, more spiritual analysis of wave phenomena in which a continuous impulse generates forms in a constantly moving medium such as water.

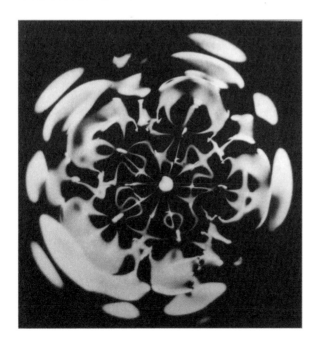

Pattern of flowers caused by vibration. From the book Kymatik by Hans Jenny (AT Verlag: Baden, 2009).

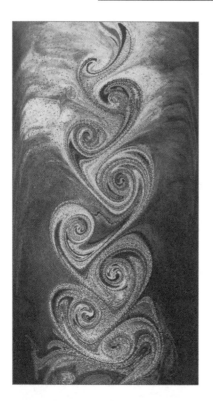

The different patterns of movement when streaming water enters recumbent water. In this photo, the water streaming in has to pass a resistance (in this case, a wide bar). This shows that when there is resistance, there is no symmetry. From the book Das sensible Chaos by Theodor Schwenk (Verlag Freies Geistesleben: Stuttgart, 2010), used with permission. This book is available in English under the title Sensitive Chaos.

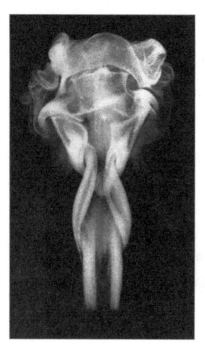

This image, which looks like a bone, was formed by water flowing into still water. When no resistance is present, symmetry is created. From the book Das sensible Chaos by Theodor Schwenk (Verlag Freies Geistesleben: Stuttgart, 2010), used with permission. This book is available in English under the title Sensitive Chaos.

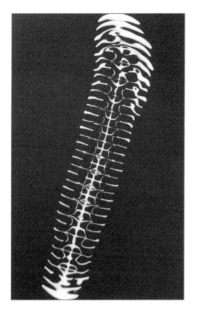

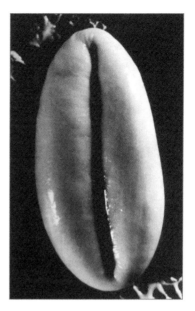

Continuous form pattern. From the book Kymatik *by Hans Jenny (AT Verlag: Baden, 2009).*

Moving three-dimensional shapes unfolding. From the book Kymatik *by Hans Jenny (AT Verlag: Baden, 2009).*

Alfred A. Tomatis

From here the trail leads to the previously mentioned French otolaryngologist Alfred A. Tomatis (1920–2001), a pioneer in sound therapy. His findings, sometimes rejected by experts, arose in a more compassionate spirit of scientific research. He came to the conclusion that there is no such thing as autism—that this is an invention of psychologists. Tomatis theorized that these children cannot access certain frequency ranges and thus they no longer hear them.

A famous example of a supposedly autistic child is the French actor Gerard Depardieu. His parents fought frequently and loudly when he was a child. In response, young Gerard dimmed his mother's screeching frequencies and his father's roaring bass until he barely felt them anymore. Over the course of many discussions, Tomatis succeeded in building a relationship of trust with Depardieu, and he gently returned him back to the world of hearing and feeling in contact with people through the use of certain sound frequencies. Tomatis saw autism as the response of the soul to unbearable noise. If the bright sound of the mother's voice is unbearable and the father's deep voice is threatening, there's not much sound world left when a child tunes out these frequencies. If the child's outside world is too painful, he builds an inner world, albeit one that is lonely and sealed off.

In working with his clients, Tomatis would use music by Mozart, certain Gregorian chants, and, if possible, a voice recording of the person's mother, which he adapted by means of an "electronic ear" he had developed, which was transmitted through special headphones. He explained that Mozart's music was not "cosmic" in the sense of being esoteric but rather that the intervals and repetitive patterns of the composer's music activate certain mental and spiritual centers in, on, and around people. He showed through his meticulous work that we can indeed regain lost skills and begin to hear again.

Alexander Lauterwasser

German researcher and photographer Alexander Lauterwasser (1951–) is particularly sensitive to the creative aspect of music. He believes that all living things in their multifarious forms embody oscillations, as expressed even in ancient texts like the Old Testament and the Indian Vedas. As the Rig Veda says, "There was neither death nor immortality then. There was no distinguishing sign of night nor of day. That one breathed, windless, by its own impulse."[2] The Creation myths of the world's peoples bear witness to the power of sound to create matter.

Here the question arises as to how the leopard comes to have its distinctive pattern of spots. Consider the figure of sound generated at a frequency of 10,101 hertz, and we can see a striking resemblance between the spots on the leopard's coat and the pattern generated by vibration.

Continuing in this vein, we discover that much slower frequencies, around 1,000 to 2,000 hertz, generate the pattern of a turtle's shell. The turtle, of course, is not known for its speed, unlike the leopard, which can strike quickly.

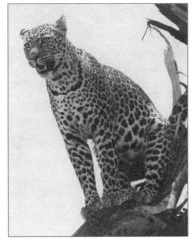

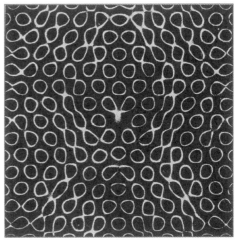

The leopard, a symbol of
strength and speed

A 10,101-hertz vibration pattern,
a very rapid oscillation

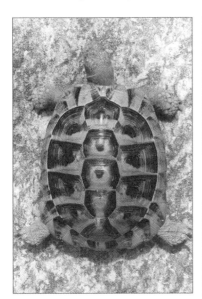

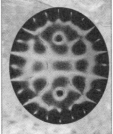

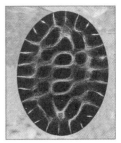

1,021-hertz
vibration pattern

2,041-hertz
vibration pattern

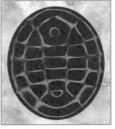

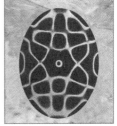

A turtle with its characteristic
armored surface

1,088-hertz
vibration pattern

1,085-hertz
vibration pattern

Significantly slower vibration patterns between 1,000 and 2,000 hertz
form a longitudinal axis with symmetrical sides.
Photos by Alexander Lauterwasser from his book Wasser, Klang, Bilder
(AT Verlag: Aarau, 2002).

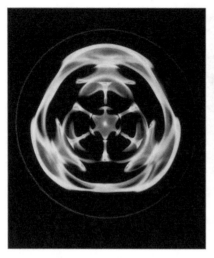 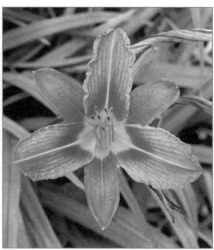

"Standing wave" with bipolar triangular structure, 28.9 hertz. Photo by Alexander Lauterwasser from his book Wasser, Klang, Bilder *(AT Verlag: Aarau, 2002).*

A lily featuring 2 bipolar 3-fold petals

Continuing, we come to the plant world. Flowers that delight us with their beauty and bright colors also carry their respective patterns, which in turn manifest as very deep, very slowly oscillating waves.

The shape shown here is born of a "standing wave"; that is, a pulsating wave vibrating in place, up and down, without moving toward our eyes, as is the case with an ocean wave. This phenomenon arises from the penetration of two opposite but similar waves.

Hans Cousto

All living things on this planet are connected by vibration. Our journey next takes us to Swiss mathematician and musicologist Hans Cousto (1948–), who discovered the natural law of the "cosmic octave" as the link between planets and sound according to mathematical rules. The rotation of our Earth causes our sleep-awake rhythm, Earth's orbit of the sun, and the growth cycles of nature. That is why it is much more life enhancing to turn artificially produced vibrations to natural vibrations.

Cousto as well as all the other pioneers whose work I mention only briefly here have been inspired by the natural order as revealed through the observation of nature. Another pioneer of this idea was Viktor Schauberger (1885–1958), who recognized the pull, the attraction, as a much more effective force and effect principle. Instead of our pressure-built technologies, he implemented nature in his own inventions. The reason why the work of Chladni has been so fascinating and why he was received by the most diverse people with enthusiasm might be because he has shown us something that lies within each one of us: the ability to create something with our actions, to build a natural order. If we continue to think along these lines we will realize that this is not only true of a violin bow but also when we speak! Furthermore, even if we do nothing at all and merely exist, we are still each a vibration that moves in the world and acts according to its form. In short, all life vibrates and generates sound, and all life has the ability to hear sound. This can be summarized as:

- Energy = Vibration = Life
- All life vibrates and generates sound.
- All life has the ability to hear sound.

Masaru Emoto

At this point enters the author of *The Message of Water,* Dr. Masaru Emoto (1943–2014), whose bestselling book showed people how vibrations affect water through his striking images of frozen water crystals. With these images he impressively demonstrated how our thoughts, words, and intentions shape matter, in this case, water. Emoto created his images of water crystals by allowing water to freeze in a cold chamber and photographing this process. It was found that the better the water quality was, the more clearly structured the crystals were, and when the water was tainted by chemicals and industrial pollution, only rough and usually incomplete crystals emerged. He expanded his research by "informing" the water with certain thoughts and words. It was found that words of beauty and love create clear, well-structured

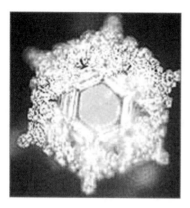

Love and gratitude.
Photo by Masaru Emoto.

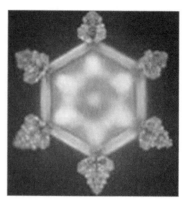

Eternity.
Photo by Masaru Emoto.

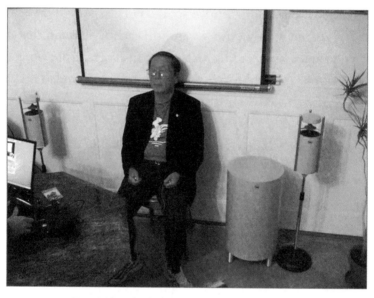

Masaru Emoto listens to the music of Mozart,
which he loved greatly. Photo by Fotolia.

crystals, while words of pain, hate, or envy had the same effect as when the water was physically contaminated.[3]

I met the extraordinary Dr. Emoto in October 2010. After a touching water-healing ritual on Lake Lucerne in Switzerland, a small group of us spent a weekend with Dr. Emoto, who spoke about his work and his way of looking at the world. He was especially hurt when other scientists dismissed his work as esoteric and unscientific, with the argument that his crystal experiments were unique and not reproducible. One can clearly see that each new crystal coming from the same source always looks a little bit different, so no general conclusions could be drawn according to his critics. This argument would be as if we all looked at one another and concluded that since each human being looks unique and very different from any other human, it cannot be that we humans have emerged from the same structures and processes. Dr. Emoto, however, had not lost his sense of humor and his curiosity. I am grateful to have met this steadfast researcher.

Is There a Connection between Memory and Hearing?

Hearing is a primary evolutionary sense in all living things. Every being is connected with everything that surrounds it through vibration. Even the simplest cell must be able to decide what enters its domain, what nourishment to accept, what it rejects, and with "whom" it wants to communicate and connect. For that to happen, the cell needs to be able to open or close, depending on the situation.

In the same way, every perception is based on information that on the physical level is always vibration. Each food particle, each molecule, all matter is, as we know from research, not fixed and static but of a certain vibration. Sound expresses this very clearly. With sound, it is not physical matter that penetrates us but a frequency that permeates us. Through the sounds that surround us we are connected to our entire environment from the very beginning. We've all had this basic experience in our mother's womb. We heard long before we saw. The control center of our physical system, the brain, has developed a great capacity for hearing. Unlike vision, we have to process what we hear right away for our own safety. If I don't hear the crackling of a dry branch under the paws of the creeping tiger, I may have to learn this lesson again in the next incarnation.

Sometimes, however, we lose touch with what surrounds us.

Alzheimer's disease is regarded as an organic brain disease. It is named after the German neurologist Alois Alzheimer (1864–1915), who first described the disease in 1906. Alzheimer's involves memory and orientation disorders, speech disorders, thinking and judgment disorders, and personality changes.[4] Consider this description of this disease from the perspective of the hearing process. As with autism, there's also a retreat from the world. There is perceived pain regarding what was heard by the person concerned, and with Alzheimer's disease, the person disconnects from the world by forgetting.

Could it be that the reason for the increasing difficulty of communicating with the world and finding your way around it is not some form of physical degeneration but instead an expression of a deeper emotional issue of the soul? When we hear, we want to fully understand what we've heard, which means that we must fully process the sound information at the level of the brain. Sometimes what you hear is painful. Aging people often no longer experience the respect that comes from fulfilling work and a sense of purpose. Also, a perceived pain means that I no longer am fully processing information, that there are gaps in what I hear. If I do not understand a piece of information entirely because I did not hear it fully, then I'm missing the big picture. Access to experiences or memories that are always connected to the hearing process remain incomplete—and what I do not understand, I also cannot remember well. For example, try reproducing a mathematical problem from school that you didn't quite understand then. On the other hand, I can well remember a connection that I have understood. Each mnemonic creates a connection, because that's how our brain works: it creates links that I can better recall.

The aspect of "bad hearing" in conjunction with forgetfulness is usually neglected. Children especially are often labeled "dense" or "stupid," when in reality they cannot fully hear and therefore also cannot fully process what they hear. This kind of situation, of course, can occur in adults too. Let us remember that the hearing process is also food for the brain, because it is powered by electrical signal transmissions.[5]

Therefore, if we can't hear, our brain isn't getting a workout. And if we don't get everything right away, we try to figure out as best we can by piecing together the rest, which leads to overload and confusion. And as with all overloads, the harder we try, the more we become disempowered in the process, because it's increasingly difficult to get the complete picture.

We often don't recognize difficulties that arise in the beginning (with hearing or other in areas). We exist in our own world, and in a sense that world is always complete. We don't know what we are missing until we experience the difference. Only when I completely hear do I realize, "Oh, there's still a lot more I can perceive, process, and experience." However, I have to know what's going on in the big picture; otherwise, with only limited information, I might think, *It's simply so, so I'll resign myself. That's just how I am.* But that doesn't have to be the case. A hearing deficit is not immutable, as we shall soon see.

5

The MUNDUS Method of Regenerating Hearing

The Step-by-Step Process

WE COME NOW TO **MUNDUS,** the basic method of hearing regeneration, the linchpin of our work. It can be used by anyone and provides information on 1) your current hearing status, 2) the coordination between your hearing and your brain, and 3) your spatial orientation. MUNDUS is the start of a step-by-step training program that will allow you to learn to hear in a more comprehensive and conscious way.

> **MUNDUS:** The name of my company, which is the organizational and economic framework for my work. The Latin word *mundus* means "world," "universe," "world order," and "cosmos"; it is the whole of heaven, earth, sea, and air as our experiential world, the world perceived by the senses, the *mundus sensibilis.* By extension, this includes the idea of a world or comprehensive cosmic order that is detectable by the intellect, or *mundus intelligibilis.*

The training described in this chapter is phase 1 of the training. Phase 2 of the MUNDUS training consists of exercises done at home between the phase 1 trainings, and these are described in the next chapters.

For phase 1 of the training you can choose your preferred sound source: either a natural sound source such as running water or a sound source consisting of music played through the Naturschallwandler natural sound transducer, both as described in chapter 1. The underlying principles of auditory processing and the construction of the listening field are equally valid for both sound sources. With the natural sound source, progress may not be as fast as with the natural sound transducer, but you will still get to your goal using running water as your sound source. However, there are differences in the practical application and the effects of these sources:

- The natural sound source of water creates a relatively uniform sound that is not easily adjusted in terms of volume. If we need a higher volume in the case of a hearing impairment, a faucet has acoustic limits (although there are ways to enhance the volume and the pitch, which I'll get into shortly).

- Sound reproduction through the Naturschallwandler natural sound transducer allows us to work with the human voice, with all its varied dynamics. Through the process of holographic reproduction, we can go right into the sound space, as if we were sitting in the middle of the orchestra in a concert hall. This experience and the related order momentum of our perception is not possible when using the sound of the water faucet or some other stationary source.

- The sound of a harmonious song and beautiful music has a pronounced effect on us. With the Naturschallwandler natural sound transducer we can also hear the sounds of everyday life while watching TV or listening to music. To do this as often as possible allows us to train our sense of hearing also.

I will now walk you through the basic therapeutic method. In the course of these instructions you will encounter some information that you have already encountered (and practiced) in chapter 1, in the first exercise, "How Well Do I Hear?" Repeating this exercise here is a way of further reifying our approach and considering the exercise more tangibly.

To assess your hearing status you will need a partner and a sound source. For the sound source you can choose either a single natural, static sound source such as the sound of running tap water, or a fountain, or the Naturschallwandler natural sound transducer described in chapter 1.

TRAINING LOCATION TO REBUILD ORDER

Let's recall that the ultimate purpose of the basic method of hearing regeneration is to become aware of how we *actually* hear and to train the entire body-mind-spirit system so that it can regulate hearing. It does not mean hearing right or better but rather training our perception of our current state: *It's on.* Now I hear *just like that.* In the course of this process you will begin to adjust your perception of hearing through the guided movements described here by aligning and balancing your body geometry. In time you will find your center. From this middle or center you will be able to regulate your hearing. Above all, your system will begin to consciously locate sound on the basis of your current perception: *Where do I hear the sound?* Through this step-by-step method of training, repeated again and again, your system will progressively learn to rebuild and improve its natural hearing ability.

"I Understood Everyone in the Circle!"

Mrs. B., 76 years old, told me, "I understood every comment, Mr. Stucki."

"Everyone *in the conversation circle?"*

Mrs. B.: "Yes, all the participants. I understood what each person said. I was completely blown away. Can you imagine?"

"This is phenomenal. I can only express my respect for how much you have worked and how well you have done."

Mrs. B.: "I'm doing the exercises that you have shown me. Now, even when I turn around, I can still hear. This used to not be the case. Before, when I turned away from the speaker in the center of the discussion circle, the voice would just go away. I'm in bliss! I feel quieter and safer within myself. All this is reflected in my spiritual life. I have a new sense of security toward life."

The Basic Therapeutic Method Using a Natural Sound Source

The question often arises as to whether we can use other natural sources of sound besides the water faucet; for example, a gong or a singing bowl. There's nothing wrong with these other sources; however, for our work it's important to have a *continuously* audible frequency spectrum, which is always the case with flowing water, as its rippling sound produces different frequencies. At the same time, repeatability and the characteristic of radiation from a single point are of importance.

Any sound not coming from a conventional speaker is considered a natural sound. There is also the sound of a jackhammer, which is not coming from a speaker; however, it seems fairly obvious that we should work with harmonious noises as much as possible. The ideal natural sound source would be a waterfall. In it we find everything from very low to very high notes, which allow us to learn through diverse vibrations that echo in very different areas of our body. Surely this is one reason why the ancient sages liked to sit at a waterfall or a flowing river. And if you want to create an even more intense experience you can enter the waterfall and let cool water splash down on you. A similar, though milder, effect can be obtained by standing in the shower.

So here we will be working with running tap water. As before, in the descriptions of these exercises the primary person undergoing training will be called the *listener,* and the helper the *partner.*

Preparation: Installation of a Therapeutic Listening Field

Set up the therapeutic seat in front of the water faucet as described in the exercise in chapter 1, page 42. If you work with a different natural sound source, the same explanations apply.

Note to Hearing Aid Users

The determination of the listener's current hearing status is best carried out without a hearing aid. With a fair amount of hearing loss, depending on the degree of loss, the exercise should be explained in detail and should, if needed, include an agreed-upon hand signal for volume control prior to the removal of the hearing aid. If the person being tested cannot understand anything without wearing the hearing aid, even very loud speaking, then the entire test should be performed with the hearing aid. In such a case the training should proceed according to the instructions in this book, but over a longer period of time before testing again without a hearing aid.

Assess Your Hearing

Please follow the exercise "How Well Do I Hear?" in chapter 1, pages 41 through 56 to assess your hearing. This simple exercise is performed only once to obtain a first-time common base for the person whose hearing is being tested. If you've already taken this test, you can continue to the next step.

Documentation and Notes

Please keep track of the maximum time for training, including the exact start time. The training should be completed after 18 to 20 minutes. To enable the partner to document the current situation and any changes, he or she should use the templates on page 133. Make a few copies of each template of the body geometry.

Preparation for the Training

You should start the next step directly after taking the test to assess your hearing. It's good to take at least a 20-minute break between sessions, but arrange a next session, if needed.

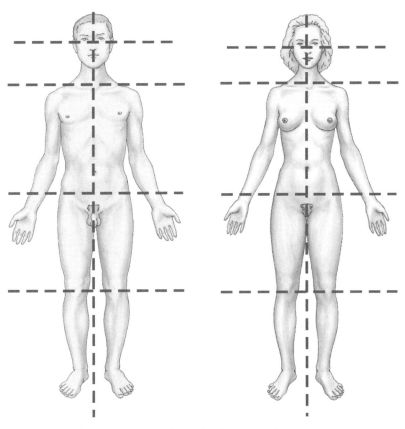

*Body geometry templates for documentation purposes
without labels for the axes*

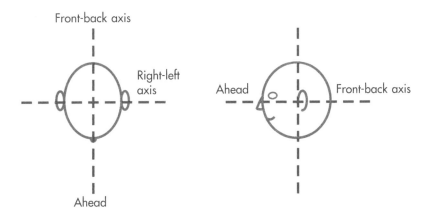

*Template for determining the position of the
sound of water in the listening field*

To prepare for the next step consider the following:

- For therapeutic training work, the listener (who is either male or female, but for the sake of brevity in these descriptions we'll refer to her as a "she" and the partner as a "he") will put on dark glasses so that she can concentrate completely on her sense of hearing. Her eyes can remain open under the dark glasses. You can also use a blindfold if that is preferable, or the listener can simply close her eyes.

- In the course of training, a fixed eye cover (either dark glasses or a blindfold) is essential for zeroing in on the sense of hearing. However, as always, it is most important that the listener feels safe, so if necessary she can remove her eye cover at any time if she feels uncomfortable.

- During training, the listener will be led between two positions in the listening field.

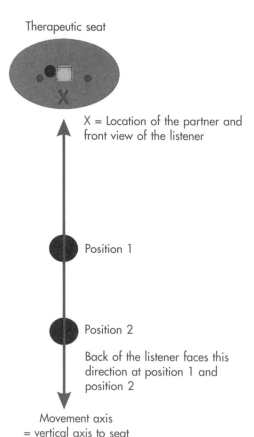

Therapeutic seat

X = Location of the partner and front view of the listener

Position 1

Position 2

Back of the listener faces this direction at position 1 and position 2

Movement axis
= vertical axis to seat

The therapeutic seat shown is with the Naturschallwandler natural sound transducer and satellites, but the idea is to give an overview of the motion axis and listening positions.

- The listener and the partner should go through the training either barefoot or in socks. This significantly strengthens the listener's body perception and substantially facilitates self-regulation, while it increases the partner's sensitivity and perception of the listener. If you want to wear shoes, they should be flat and as soft as possible, such as ballet shoes or slippers.

- Before starting, the partner asks whether it is okay to align the shoulder and head axes of the listener by means of contact, should this be necessary. Proper alignment of the body geometry is key to building a proper hearing perception and to improving hearing.

- The aim of training is for the listener to correctly identify the location of the sound source (both the running water and the sound of the partner's voice) on the vertical axis from the front. There are two different listening positions along the vertical axis, each having a different distance from the therapeutic seat, according to the sketch above. If the listener is able to orient from where the sound is coming, she is led to the therapeutic seat and seated so that the sound source is behind her.

- When the listening position changes, the sound source should be clearly and unambiguously heard from behind. This is the natural and correct spatial auditory perception position in the therapeutic seat.

Again, the training described here is training phase 1. Phase 2 training is the training between the trainings, the exercises carried out by the person at home.

Explanation for the Companion

The goal at this stage is for the listener to try to locate the direction of the sound source clearly and unambiguously first from the front. Ideally this exercise will be carried out while both the listener as well as the partner are standing. If the person, however, feels uncertain in this position, this phase can be done seated. In this case, a chair with wheels, such as an office chair or a wheelchair, can be used so that the listener can move without having to get up.

Make sure that the listener and you (if you are the partner) can move freely on the vertical axis, preferably toward the wall opposite the therapeutic seat.

Training Phase 1, Part 1

Follow these step-by-step instructions:

- The listener stands on the front-back axis facing the therapeutic seat at a distance of about 1.5 to 2.5 yards. This is the first listening position in the sketch, position 1.
- The listener puts on the dark glasses. It is important that the sides of the glasses are positioned above the ears. The glasses should fit firmly but not too tightly. The eyes can be open or closed under the glasses during the entire exercise—whatever is more pleasant for the person. Alternatively, the listener can wear a blindfold.
- The partner turns on the tap slightly so that the sound of the

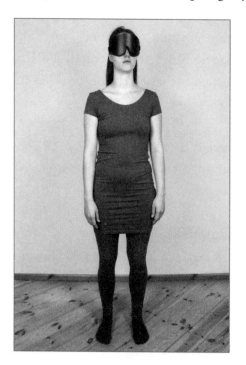

The person may feel comfortable, but the body alignment is wrong: her right shoulder axis is sloping and the left shifted back; the right hand rests significantly lower than the left hand, and the head is turned to the left axis.

running water can just be heard. The partner should ask the listener to stand comfortably. Note that the partner doesn't ask the listener to stand straight.

- The partner pays attention to how the listener is standing in terms of her body axes and also takes note of her stance. As long as it's been agreed on in advance, the partner takes a picture of the listener to record the position of her body.
- The position of the listener's body axes is drawn according to the template.
- The partner turns up the tap a little more and asks, "Can you clearly hear the sound of water?"
- As long as the listener does not clearly hear the water noise, the partner continues to slowly turn up the volume of water coming out in the faucet until the listener can hear the sound clearly.
- The sound volume of the water can be amplified by placing a prop such as a pot (or something else "tinny" that amplifies the sound)

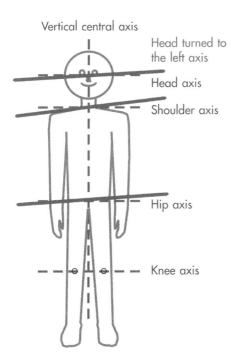

Example sketch of the body axes

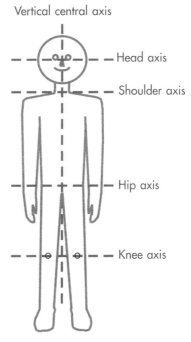

Blank template of the body axes

right-side up or upside down under the faucet. Please have a prop like this handy in case you need to make the noise louder.

- A low sound volume during the test doesn't result in strengthening but serves more as a burden. The person might be able to hear the running water but can't hear it loud enough for their comfort level. In that case the volume should be adjusted accordingly, because as the training progresses, the hearing threshold will gradually improve.

- All questions are always asked by the partner in the same position as the listener. For example, if the listener is seated, then the partner should also sit. If the listener is standing, the partner stands directly in front of her and asks questions from that position. In this way the front-back axis for the training is always respected.

Training Phase 1, Part 2

Follow these step-by-step instructions:

- The partner now asks the listener to move back and forth (the direction started does not matter) with the whole body, including the feet, once to the left with up to 90 degrees deviation from the main axis, then once to the right with up to 90 degrees deviation from the main axis. (The listener should not leave the standing position).

- By further oscillating, the listener is seeking alignment with the sound source. She should oscillate until she clearly hears it from the front. Thus the current orientation of the person is determined regarding the alignment of the entire body to the sound source. This shows how much the hearing differs from the center.

- The person should not just turn her head but should instead align her entire body to the sound source.

- If the person is not exactly standing on the front-back axis but has a shifted alignment to the sound source, you will now help her align on the front-back axis. For this purpose, grasp the listener firmly but gently on the shoulders, and turn her carefully until the upper body and head are again aligned exactly in the direction of the sound source. Usually the person follows this movement with their feet.

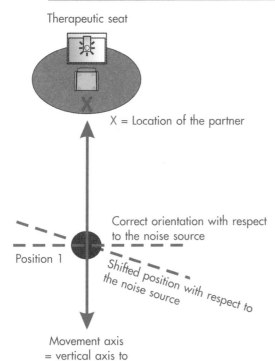

Therapeutic seat

X = Location of the partner

Correct orientation with respect to the noise source

Position 1

Shifted position with respect to the noise source

Movement axis = vertical axis to the seat position

Check the alignment for the noise source (the running water coming from the sink shown in this picture).

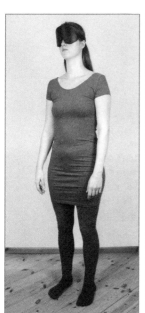

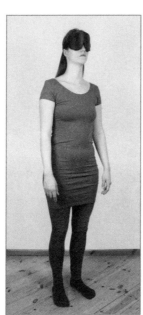

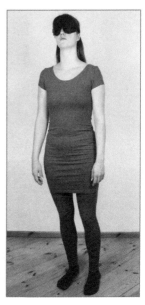

Turn to the right as shown, on the axis.

Turn to the left, on the axis.

Turn back toward the center, not quite as much as the first time.

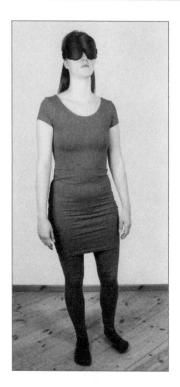

Turn back in the other direction. The listener should move using a pendulum motion until she feels that she is exactly facing the sound source.

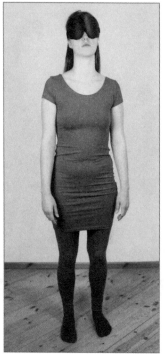

The listener is using her auditory perception to align with the sound source, until the sound source is exactly in front of her (actually in the picture, however, the orientation is shifted to the left).

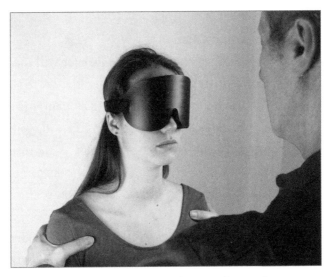

Orient the listener to the sound source by gently rotating her shoulders so that they are perpendicular to the source.

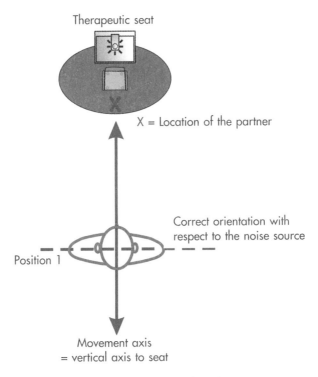

The listener is correctly oriented to the noise source (possibly after an adjustment by the partner).

Training Phase 1, Part 3

Follow these step-by-step instructions:

- We pause for about 20 seconds, then the listener will move for the first time on the front-back axis.

- Gently grasp the listener by the shoulders. By gently pressing the shoulder of the listener backward and then forward, you will find the right direction in which this movement is performed—the direction in which the person moves easily is the correct one. If you are unsure of which direction it is, lead the person backward or farther away from the sound source.

- The partner moves the listener carefully but with confidence in the correct direction and then stops her. Then, without letting go, he moves the listener's upper body to the right and then to the left a few more times, gently swaying back and forth, to give her an opportunity to calmly juxtapose her feet and realign herself.

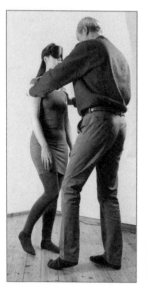 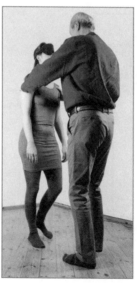 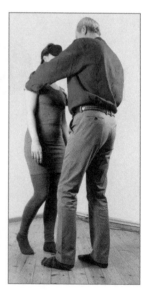

The partner leads by using a pulsating pressure lightly on the shoulders of the listener in the desired direction while they both move together.

Lead with small steps.

One more step.

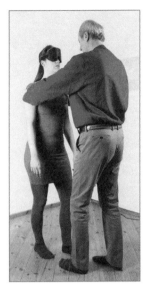

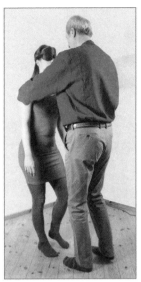

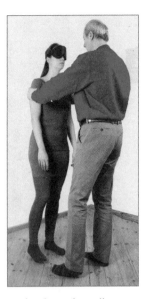

Gently stop to offset the feet.	*By applying lateral pressure in the correct direction, you give the listener an opportunity to juxtapose her feet with yours.*	*This lateral oscillating movement is smoothly executed so that the listener can lift her other foot and align herself easily. This movement also relaxes the body.*

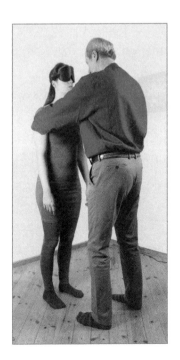

The listener is reoriented after the movement in the direction of the noise source. All photos of this aspect of the exercise by Jutta Ebinger.

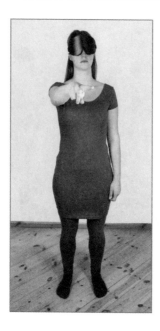

The listener shows where in the room she hears the sound.

- At this point the partner returns to where the therapeutic seat is located and asks, "Where do you hear the sound of water? Please indicate with your hand, no matter where you hear it."
- With an outstretched arm, the listener points to where she perceives the sound. This gives you information about the accuracy of her spatial orientation with respect to the sound source.
- This third part of the training phase 1 is repeated several times until the person can hear the running water reasonably clearly from the front area. With a strong hearing imbalance, it is sufficient that the noise is heard from the front; it doesn't have to be displayed precisely in the center.
- In addition to trying to locate the sound of the water noise, the listener will also indicate from which direction she hears her partner's voice when the partner asks, "Where do you hear me? Where am I? Please indicate with your hand, no matter where that is."
- The partner keeps repeating this question until the listener has found the direction of the partner's voice and indicates it correctly by pointing with an outstretched arm. This may be different from

the actual position of the water noise source, or it might be in the same place. This makes it easier for you as a partner to develop a feel for how the correction process is going. The listener can then also determine how good the fine-tuning of their hearing is in terms of trying to locate two different sound sources, both the water noise and the partner's voice.

- The partner's repeated question regarding his or her own position adds a second impulse to strengthen sound source orientation. The listener's perception of the position of the partner is often more accurate than the perception of the water noise, because the partner always comes to the listener from the front and establishes physical contact. Thus the partner provides a constant for the listener in terms of orienting herself, unlike the water noise, which is only sound in the room and can be located only through auditory perception.

Note to the Partner: Aligning Body Geometry

For the success of the basic method, it is crucial that the body geometry of the person is properly aligned. This means that the head position (the head axis) and/or the shoulder axis of the listener should be aligned by the partner and, if necessary, corrected. Alignment means that the head and shoulder axes are parallel to each other and at the same time at right angles to the front-back axis. You, the partner, are responsible for this alignment and for doing it in such a way that the listener does not get frightened. The first contact with your hands is always the same on both the right and the left upper arms of the listener, near her shoulders. You should guide her gently and surely and slowly align her body. This intervention has a strong effect and must be carried out with sensitivity to the listener, because a change in the usual posture can sometimes be irritating for some people.

The position of the hands for aligning the listener's upper body is the same as for moving her around in the room. If the shoulders change their alignment after the head has been aligned—which is not unusual—then do not correct the shoulders, as the overall body geometry is always determined by the head geometry.

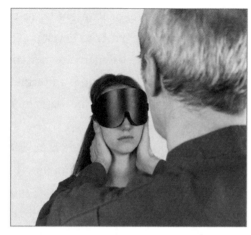

Gently align the head.

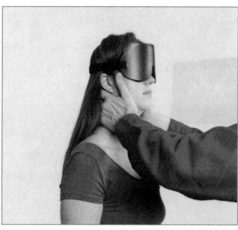

Alignment of the head from a lateral perspective. Photos of this aspect of the exercise by Jutta Ebinger.

Correction of the person's posture and body geometry, especially the orientation of the head, is especially important if the position of the water noise is not found unambiguously from the front and/or if the head position is lopsided, as often happens with weak hearing. People usually position their head so that the stronger ear faces forward. However, in this position the head is not clearly aligned to the sound source, making it hard to correct the difficulty in finding location of the sound source.

If it is not possible to touch the listener (because she doesn't want to be touched or you don't want to touch her), the correction can be done verbally. For example, the partner might say, "Please turn your head slightly to the right" if the listener's head geometry is off (just remember that your right is the person's left, and vice versa). Or, for instance, to adjust the height of the shoulders you might say, "Please relax the right shoulder and lift the left shoulder a bit." Try not to make more than 2 or 3 corrections in a training session of 20 minutes, because too many corrections made in succession can make the listener feel insecure.

For developing balanced body geometry during the times between training sessions, the mirror exercise described in chapter 2 (pages 70 through 75) is recommended.

Training Phase 1, Part 4

Follow these step-by-step instructions:

- If the listener can clearly identify the direction of the running water upon first try, then a milestone has been reached.
- The next training step will be to have the listener clearly identify, from different positions, the location of the running water as coming from the front at least twice in a row. To do the training, follow the procedure from phase 1, part 3 to move the listener into different positions on the front-back axis and test them from these alternate positions.
- If this fails or takes too long (the total time of the training session should be no more than 20 minutes), then you should stop the exercise and try again after 1 to 3 days have passed.

Pausing or Ending at Phase 1, Part 4

- Go to the faucet and turn it off slowly. Then go to the listener and put a chair behind her, so that the front edge of the chair lightly touches the back of her legs. Tell her that the chair is directly behind her and help her sit down by gently but securely grasping her upper arms as you guide her.
- Once she is seated, go over to the therapeutic seat and sit down as well. Then tell the listener, "Please take off your dark glasses slowly."

- Ask her how she feels and what she experienced. If a lot has happened, give her enough time to discuss her experience completely.
- If the training is complete for the day, see the instructions titled "Downtime" (page 151).

Note: When the Sound "Jumps"

In all stages of training it is possible that the perception of the position of the water noise jumps sharply. For example, the listener hears the noise only from the side, then from the front, then possibly from behind. This can occur especially when a new position on the front-back axis is taken. This jumping phenomenon may also apply to the location of the partner's voice; however, this is more rare.

This sudden jump is a good sign, and the listener needs to be assured that this is so. It is a clear signal that the person has modified their usual hearing pattern and their system is looking for a new order. As I have said, in the beginning it's not important to be right, because with time and continued training the new order becomes set.

Training Phase 1, Part 5

Follow these step-by-step instructions:

- During the course of training, if the listener can hear the sound of the running water from the front from two different positions, then lead her to the area in front of the faucet while the water is still running.
- Make sure that the position to where you lead her is not too far from the therapeutic seat, as "blind" walking in itself is a challenge. In this case, on the way to therapeutic seat ask the listener again, "Where do you hear the sound of water coming from? Please indicate with your hand, no matter where that is." As I said, it's not about getting to the seat quickly but about building a stable and well-established space with the correct positioning of the sound sources.
- Guide the listener to the therapeutic seat and slowly turn her

180 degrees to the right so she's standing with her back to the seat. Ask her to sit down, gently stabilizing her by grasping her upper arms to support and secure her.

- At the conclusion of this process, a full adjustment of the auditory perception will occur (i.e., the adjustment of the reference point at the back of the head in connection with the fully balanced body geometry). The water noise, which has been heard from various positions relative to the therapeutic seat, is now clearly perceived from behind by the listener sitting in therapeutic seat. This creates a clear reference point for acoustic perception in the listening field.

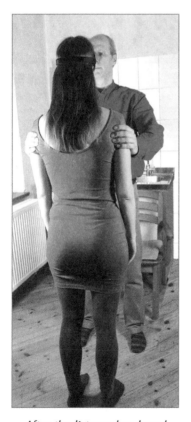 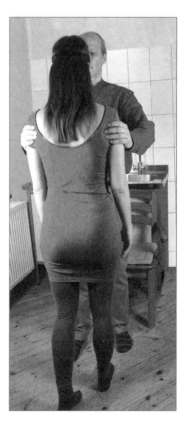

After the listener has heard the sound source correctly from the front 2 times in a row, guide the listener to the therapeutic seat by gently grasping her shoulders.

Move her toward the seat.

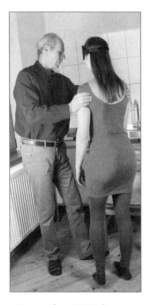

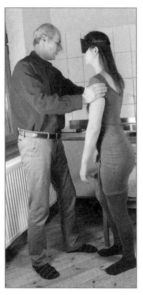

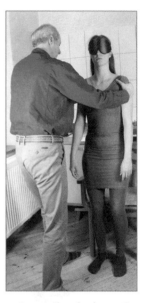

Rotate her 180 degrees (clockwise or counterclockwise) in front of the seat.

Turn her gently but firmly, in one smooth motion, without releasing her shoulders.

Rotate her body until she is standing in front of the seat.

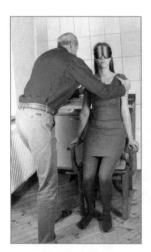

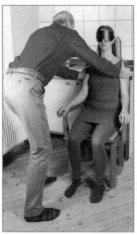

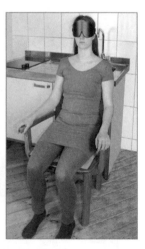

The listener continues to be held by her shoulders as she sits down in the chair.

Gently grasping her shoulders, assist her in sitting down until she is comfortably resting against the back of the chair. Photos of this aspect of the exercise by Jutta Ebinger.

The listener now sits relaxed in the seat and can hear the sound of the running water directly behind her.

Training Phase 1, Part 6: At the Sound Source

Follow these step-by-step instructions:

- The listener sits relaxed in the chair. Slowly turn the tap off.
- Sit down at a distance of about 2 yards from her, facing her.
- Tell her she can now slowly take off the dark glasses, and give her some time.
- Please remain vigilant; monitor and record her reactions; for example, her complexion, expression, state of relaxation, and mood.
- After you've turned off the water, ask her where she heard the sound of the running water coming from last. After that, ask her how she feels and what her experience was like. It is important that she shares everything that she feels at this moment.

Downtime

Before the final debriefing, give the listener a few minutes to process the total experience in silence.

As a partner in this process, ensure that there is protected and undisturbed downtime. If a lot has happened, give her time to process internally.

Debriefing

Looking back, discuss the basic method in which a natural sound source was used. What did the listener experience? What did you perceive as a partner? Be restrained and sensitive, and allow the listener to reflect. As the partner in this process it makes sense to communicate to the listener *your* observations regarding her movements and posture during the exercise, including any changes in the volume of water noise. In this way the listener is supported in perceiving how much the listening field was in motion and that she built this listening field herself.

Discuss the following points:

- Results and observations of the training that has just been carried out

- Additional actions.
- Schedule the next training dates.
- Confirm the exercises to do at home until the next training session to strengthen and further support the listening field. First and foremost for this kind of "homework" is the mirror exercise described in chapter 2 (pages 70 through 75). The remaining exercises, done at home, are described in the next chapters, and are considered phase 2 of training.
- Clarify any questions.

It is important to emphasize to the listener that hearing improvement is based on continuous training. Arrange a training program consisting of 3 to 10 sessions to stabilize the hearing progress and to complete the overall process.

If the perception of the position of the water noise or the sound of the partner's voice during the training moved greatly, it's important to explain that this is a very good sign showing the body is seeking a new order.

In phase 1, 2 appointments per week are ideal, with 1 to 2 days between appointments. Of course, the intervals between sessions can be longer, but not so long that what has been achieved is lost again. That's why shorter intervals are recommended in the beginning—no longer than 1 week. These can then be gradually extended.

Notes for the Partner to Complete
after the Session

- What has changed in the listener's auditory perception, in their attitude, in their sense of volume, and so on?
- Note the spatial localizations of the person if you have not already done so during the process.
- Be sure to read the "Conclusion to the Basic Method" at the end of this chapter (pages 180–181).

THE BASIS FOR THE EFFECTS OF
THE MUNDUS BASIC METHOD

Let's now review some of the key aspects of the basic method. It's important for me to explain again why we do things the way we do—because the better we understand something, the more effectively we can apply it and use it.

Listening and moving while blindfolded, the sound of the running water receives a specific location wihtin the listening field, when it is perceived by the listener. It's not important at first when the listener first hears it. It does not matter in the beginning whether her internal perceptions match the external reality; that is, whether the source of the water noise (or the sound of the partner's voice) are actually where the listener perceives them. The only important point is that the listener, without the help of her eyes, can determine the location of the sound of the running water.

By identifying where the water noise is, a reference point is established. With this, a kind of relationship is established as well, whereby the listener has to decide: "Where am I? Where are the other sources of noise?" This choice can no longer be arbitrary; the listener must define and decide where the noise source is in space. With this decision, order is established.

By deciding on a location, a process is set in motion. Listening becomes more conscious than previously, when the listening process was habitual and therefore weakened. So, I am made aware of my previous state of being, and by bringing conscious awareness to it, bit by bit I am able to process what has weakend my sense of hearing. This is accomplished at the listener's own speed, because only she can know for herself which speed is right for her.

This is the beginning of learning how to hear better, because better balance and processing of sound within the total body system will lead to better hearing.

This whole process of reorganizing how we hear can be taxing on the body and also on the brain. Remember how you once learned arithmetic, or read your first words, or formed your first letters—is the bow on the left or on the right? Or how to make a fire, use a saw, or learn a new course of study in college? Even though there may be positive memories, it was nevertheless tiring and challenging to integrate new information. In each situation or individual lesson, we could only handle a certain amount of information, and if our teachers presented us with too much information we quickly became overwhelmed.

The same is true of the basic hearing regeneration method: it's important not to go too fast and risk becoming overwhelmed. For this reason the training sessions are limited to a maximum of 20 minutes. Even if we move only a little bit during the session, seemingly doing very little, it's still tiring. As the body starts to regulate and adjust, its center of balance will become more certain. This gradual change can be a bit of a strain, because we are challenged on the mental and emotional level as well.

Every being strives to expand and grow. Sometimes there are situations, however, where these growth impulses are thwarted by physical or mental pain restrictions. During training we might encounter those situations from our past. This work causes the underlying painful content to come to light to be consciously reviewed, piece by piece. The process is similar to organizing a cabinet. Once organization takes place, the contents can be easily viewed.

This is another reason why it's very important to proceed at the pace and in the manner that's right for each person. As a partner in the process, I do not really know what is right for the listener—only she can know that. My job as a partner is to follow the lead of the listener, who is working at the speed that's right for her.

As training proceeds, the noise source may move to the center, or farther away, or up or down, sometimes even backward. Again and again I perceive the water noise, and with that perception comes the feedback, "Aha, it changes!" As this occurs, I wander through the library of my life. Many a book I touch in passing, some just for a moment, but some I have to reread carefully to remember the contents of what really happened.

Over the course of training this processing means releasing in whole or in part previously suppressed content. Here our system works like a holographic filing system wherein events, feelings, and thoughts are linked together and temporal classifications take place in which the sequence of events is clarified, experiences and events are connected for reevaluation, and new insights are drawn.

Hilde's Story: Planes Mean Death

One evening near Cologne, Germany, the following occurred in the living room of a gathering of friends and family that I attended.

In a relaxed atmosphere, I told the group about the background of hearing impairment. Almost everyone present was interested, and some sat down near the Naturschallwandler, while the rest of us observed the head and body posture of the listeners—how their ears were aligned, and the amount of sound that was pleasant for each person.

The evening was a bit advanced in terms of the steps usually taken in our training, but we proceeded anyway. The oldest person in the group, a woman named Hilde, said that she wanted to try sitting by the Naturschallwandler. She had earlier said in the round of introductions that she had been hearing a lot worse for about the past 10 years, ever since she had moved to a small house under the flight path of the Cologne airport. Since then, her hearing had decreased significantly, she said. The doctor she had consulted at one point told her that this certainly had something to do with her age and, of course, with the noise pollution from the jets arriving and taking off. She had tried hearing aids, but she couldn't handle them at all.

As she sat in the seat by the Naturschallwandler, I played, as usual, the first song by Eva Cassidy, and Hilde immediately became very restless. She insisted that I turn the volume up, as she heard and understood nothing. I told her that it would be no problem, but it could also be that the singer was singing in English, and if a language is unfamiliar it would be very difficult at times to understand what the singer was singing.

She interrupted me, a little angry, and said, "But that's not it—I was an English teacher, and I should be able to understand." She shifted uncomfortably on her seat, back and forth. My question of where she could hear the singer revealed that Hilde heard the singer forward and to the right. I saw that the situation was becoming exhausting for her and that it was difficult for her to establish a clear position of the sound. I asked her if she wanted to do a little exercise with me, and she said yes. Then I asked her to stand up and sit down opposite the listening position on a chair. I put myself at the listening position by the Naturschallwandler where she was previously seated and let the music continue to play softly. Now I asked her to simply focus on my voice and the singer's.

We went on talking about different aspects of her hearing and how close her house is from the airport and the height of the aircraft overhead. Her description revealed that the distances were actually not that close. Certainly jet aircraft don't produce beautiful sounds and can be irritating, but the direct noise exposure didn't really explain her progressive hearing loss because the planes flew at a relatively high altitude above her house.

I asked Hilde again and again to just close her eyes and listen to the singer and to show me where she could hear the singer's voice coming from. Gradually, she heard the singer and my own voice becoming clearer and clearer. After about 15 minutes I asked her again to close her eyes, and this time she very clearly pointed out that the singer was coming from the front. I then asked her to get up and go to the therapeutic seat and sit down again by the Naturschallwandler. At the same time, I got up, walked around to the place where she had been sitting, and reduced the volume so that the voice of the singer was now clear, but not loud.

When she sat down again, she clearly heard the singer behind her. She said, "Oh, this is loud now, I understand everything she is singing now!" It was very surprising for all who were present. She was very moved by this situation. Her eyes moistened as she began to speak: "I *suddenly get many pictures. I don't know where they are coming from. I see planes and low-flying aircraft from the war, when my mother was on the run with my sister and me, and my sister was injured in a low-flying attack. I feel a great fear of the planes. And now I understand why I've never felt comfortable in my house."*

Her friend said, "Hilde, we've known each other for 40 years, and you've never told me that you're afraid of airplanes."

Hilde replied, "That's right. I didn't know it—until today!"

In the past, because of perceived pain in a dangerous or threatening situation, we may have created a protective response to a perceived danger that resulted in certain mental distortions or fears. Initially this response enabled us to process the traumatic experience in some way in the here and now. Thus Hilde's fear of aircraft, with all its dangerous implications for her, had affected her hearing, which she had turned down as an adaptive response. She found, however, that she could resolve this issue. She realized that she did not have to be afraid of aircraft anymore and therefore no longer had to protect herself from them by shutting down her hearing.

Again, it should be emphasized that if we try to accelerate this self-regulation process by any form of pressure or try to force a listener into their center, the result will not be self-regulation but rather fear, uncertainty, and resistance. We must regulate, not manipulate. We don't push, we give impulses. This is the guiding principle behind our work.

The journey is the destination. That means it's all about focusing on the process, not on the results. Of course, if I am well trained and experienced, I can help someone with a strongly shifted sense of hearing into balance with a *whoosh*. This may seem great, especially if the pain recedes, but if the initial shift has occurred over a long period of time, the listener will either fall back into her well-known groove or develop other symptoms so long as the underlying trauma is not resolved.

BUILDING TRUST AND COMMUNICATION

We are all a bit blind to ourselves. That's why we need people around us. In the basic method, the partner has a very important and beautiful role, as we have seen in the exercises in this chapter: to lead the listener toward natural hearing and to be her reflection, giving her impulses for physical alignment and balance. This is actually a challenge shared by both participants.

The listener agrees to work with the partner and allows herself to be guided. For many people, this alone is already an enormous exercise in trust. And to allow oneself to be touched physically when getting aligned requires an even greater degree of trust. That's why it's absolutely important to not cross boundaries. For the listener who is blindfolded and undergoing training, it's not about persevering or enduring something that feels uncomfortable. Stopping is always better than pushing through. Not everything can or will be healed in one session, and I may not always want a stranger near me during this process.

For this reason, good communication is vital; we have to be assured that the training can be canceled at any time. Also, because it's a challenge for the partner to be clear and to provide a sense of security, both in orientating the body of the listener and in moving her, communication should be well established from the outset.

The Basic Therapeutic Method Using a Natural Sound Transducer

As noted earlier, an advantage of training using a natural sound transducer such as the Naturschallwandler is that through the holographic reproduction of sound it corresponds to the way sound behaves in nature. The method of restoring hearing naturally does not work with conventional speakers, because regardless of their sound quality they do not duplicate natural spatiality the way this holographic technology does. Once I move in front of a conventional speaker, the sound changes;

that is, it moves based on my movement. This does not correspond to how sound behaves in nature. In nature, a fixed noise source is always at its point of origin, even if I move in front of it or around it.

As before, in the descriptions of these exercises the primary person undergoing training will be called the *listener,* and the helper the *partner.*

Preparation: Installation of a Therapeutic Listening Field

Set up the therapeutic seat and the Naturschallwandler natural sound transducer system as described in chapter 1, pages 48 through 50.

Note to Hearing Aid Users

The determination of the listener's current hearing status is best carried out without a hearing aid. With a fair amount of hearing loss, depending on the degree of loss, the exercise should be explained in detail and should, if needed, include an agreed-upon hand signal for volume control prior to the removal of the hearing aid.

If the person being tested cannot understand anything without wearing the hearing aid, even very loud speaking, then the entire test should be performed with the hearing aid. In such a case the training should proceed according to the instructions in this book, but over a longer period of time before testing again without a hearing aid.

Assess Your Hearing

Please review the exercise "How Well Do I actually Hear?" in chapter 1 (pages 41 through 56).

This simple test is performed only once to obtain a base for the listener and the partner. Once you have completed this test, the basic method using a natural sound transducer such as the Naturschallwandler begins as follows.

Technology and Music

The selection of music and control of volume are done by remote control.

We use a centered female singing voice, as noted in chapter 1. We have worked with the following two songs for many years, with great success:

- Song 1: "Over the Rainbow," by Eva Cassidy, from her CD *Songbird*
- Song 2: "Spanish Harlem," by Rebecca Pidgeon, from her CD *The Raven*

For our therapeutic work we will need these two songs copied onto a single disk so we can work without having to change CDs and so we can play them on repeat with the remote control. To do this, download these songs and copy them to a disk or USB flash drive. Please make sure that the quality is not reduced by compression or error during copying.

We discussed the musical qualities of the Eva Cassidy piece in chapter 1; the second piece, by Rebecca Pidgeon, fulfills these same qualities. Pidgeon sings in a lower pitch than Cassidy, so both pieces running consecutively cover a relatively wide spectrum of sound.

We have chosen female voices for our work, as female voices cause less fear in most people. This is associated with the fact that most hearing problems are related to forms of violence, and violence usually emanates from men. If you experience these women's voices unpleasantly, pick another unique voice, even if it's male. What's paramount is that the voice is centered and clear, making it easy to locate.

Documentation and Notes

So that the partner can document the current situation and changes, he uses the following templates. Simply make a few copies.

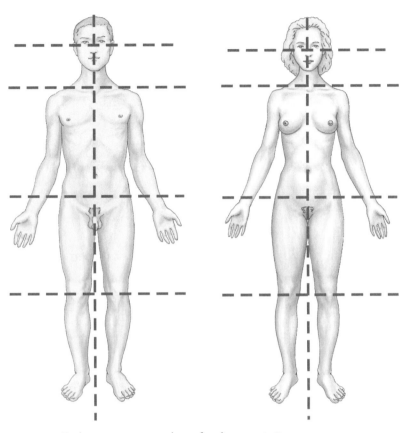

*Body geometry templates for documentation purposes,
without labels for the axes*

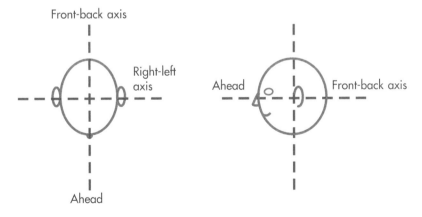

*Template for determining the position of
the singer in the room*

Preparation for the Training

You should only start the basic method of hearing regeneration directly after the initial **anamnesis,** if the person is amenable and his or her strength allows it. In any case, it's good to take a break at least every 20 minutes between the different sections of this training. And it's always better to arrange a new meeting date if necessary.

Anamnesis: a preliminary case history of a patient (Greek, *anamnesis,* "memory")

Our method includes the following:

- For therapeutic training work, the listener puts on dark glasses so that she can concentrate solely on the sense of hearing. The eyes can remain open under the glasses. You can also cover the eyes with a mask or simply close your eyes. In the course of training, a fixed eye cover for zeroing in on the sense of hearing helps to ensure success; however, as always, the point is that the listener feels safe, so they should be told ahead of time that they can remove their dark glasses or eye cover at any time if they feel uncomfortable.

- During training, the listener will be guided back and forth in the listening field between several positions.

- You should both go through this training either barefoot or in socks. This significantly strengthens one's body perception and increases sensitivity, thereby facilitating regulation. If you want to wear shoes, wear only ones without heels and as soft as possible, such as ballet shoes or slippers, which allow the feet to move naturally.

- Before starting training, the partner establishes whether it's okay for him to align the listener's shoulders and head axes by means of physical contact, should this be necessary. Proper alignment of the body geometry is a key aspect to building proper hearing perception and improving hearing.

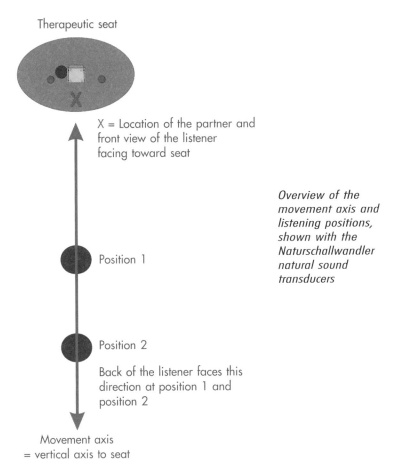

Therapeutic seat

X = Location of the partner and front view of the listener facing toward seat

Position 1

Position 2

Back of the listener faces this direction at position 1 and position 2

Movement axis = vertical axis to seat

Overview of the movement axis and listening positions, shown with the Naturschallwandler natural sound transducers

- The aim of training is that the listener should spatially hear the sound source in addition to the partner's voice. During this training exercise the partner faces the listener on the vertical axis. This exercise should be done from at least two different positions on the vertical axis that have different distances from the therapeutic seat, as shown in the figure above. If the location of the sound source is indicated correctly (that it is directly in front of the listener), the listener will be led to the therapeutic seat, turned around, and then seated.
- When the position of the listener changes at this step in training, the singer will be heard clearly from behind. This is the natural and correct spatial auditory perception in the therapeutic seat.

Again, the training described here is training phase 1. Phase 2 is the training between the trainings; that is, the exercises carried out by the person at home, which are described in later chapters.

Explanation for the Companion

The goal at this stage is for the person to be able to clearly locate the direction of sound from the front.

Ideally this identification of sound coming from the front will be carried out while standing; however, if the person feels insecure standing, this can be done seated, in which case a chair with wheels such as an office chair or wheelchair is used so that the person can move without having to get up.

Make sure that you and the person can move freely on the vertical axis, preferably toward the wall opposite the therapeutic seat.

Training Phase 1, Part 1

Follow these step-by-step instructions:

- The listener stands on the front-back axis to face the therapeutic seat at a distance of about 1.50 to 2.50 yards. This is the first listening position in the sketch, position 1.
- The listener puts on the dark glasses or eyeshade. It is important that the sides of the glasses are positioned above the ears. The glasses should sit securely but not fit too tightly. The eyes can be open or closed during the entire exercise; however, it may be more pleasant for the listener to keep her eyes open under the glasses.
- The partner takes the remote control and plays song 1 softly. Then he puts the remote control to the side, making sure to ask the listener to stand in a comfortable position. Note that the partner does not ask the listener to stand straight.
- The partner observes how the listener's posture looks in terms of body axes and takes note of her stance. If it has been agreed upon in advance, a photo is taken.
- The partner then documents the current position of her body axes on the template provided.

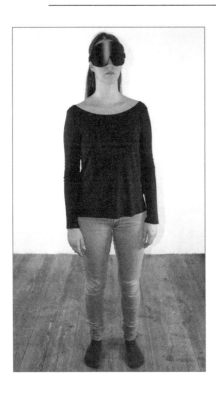

She is standing comfortably, but her body axes are clearly out of balance.

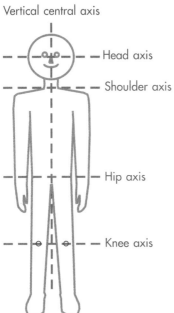

A template for recording the body axes

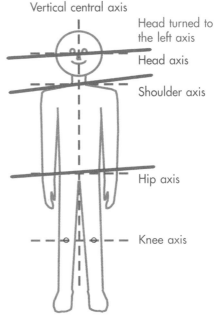

A record of the listener's body axes as seen in the photo above. Her shoulder axes are off, with her right shoulder sloping and her left shoulder shifted back. The right hand rests significantly lower than the left hand, and the head is turned toward the left axis.

- The partner then takes the remote control and increases the volume slightly, until the listener is comfortable with the volume level. Your previous verbal interactions with the listener will give an estimate of how loud the volume may need to be.

- After playing the first song, the volume is gradually increased until it reaches the same volume as during the preliminary procedure, where the listener understood everything the partner was saying. A low sound volume during the test doesn't result in strengthening but serves more as a burden. Then the partner asks, "Is the singer easy to understand?"

- The partner adjusts the volume until it is pleasing to the person, which must be confirmed by repeating the question, "Is the singer easy to understand?" Always remember that the volume level will be very high for those who are hard of hearing.

- The listener should hear the singer well, but not too loudly. Throughout training the volume should be adjusted according to the progress made since the auditory threshold should be improving.

- All questions are always asked by the partner from the position of the therapeutic seat. If the listener is sitting, the partner will also be sitting. Thus the front-back axis for the listener is always respected.

Training Phase 1, Part 2

Follow these step-by-step instructions:

- The partner now asks the listener to move back and forth on the axis (the direction in which the movement is started does not matter) with the whole body, including the feet, once to the left with up to 90 degrees deviation from the main axis, then once to the right with up to 90 degrees deviation from the main axis. (The listener should not leave the standing position).

- By oscillating back and forth like a pendulum, alignment can now be found, in which the listener has the feeling that she is directly facing the singer and the singer can be clearly heard from the front. This part of the exercise helps determine the current orientation of the listener to the sound source and how near or far away from

Therapeutic seat

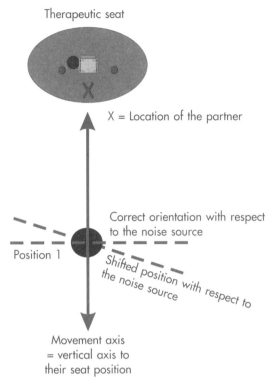

X = Location of the partner

Check the alignment to the noise source.

Correct orientation with respect to the noise source

Position 1

Shifted position with respect to the noise source

Movement axis = vertical axis to their seat position

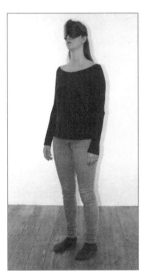

Turn to the right on the axis.

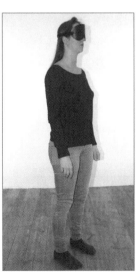

Leftward rotation on the axis

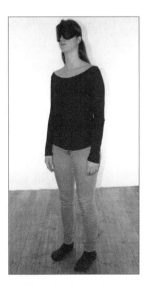

Turn back again to the other side, but not quite as much as the first time.

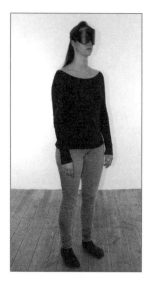

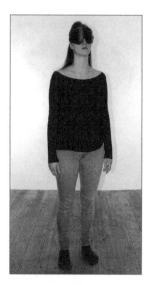

Turn back again in the other direction with a pendulum motion until the listener feels she is exactly facing the sound source.

The listener's auditory perception is now directly facing the sound source (although slightly to the left in this picture).

alignment she is. The listener needs to orient her whole body toward the sound source, not just her head. If the listener isn't standing straight on the front-back axis but is shifted in her orientation to the sound source, her alignment needs to be straightened.

- Firmly but sensitively clasp the listener by both of her shoulders and turn her until her upper body and head have returned to the sound source. Usually the listener will follow this slight adjustment with her feet.

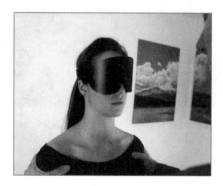

Orient the listener to the sound source by rotating her shoulders so that they are exactly perpendicular to the sound source.

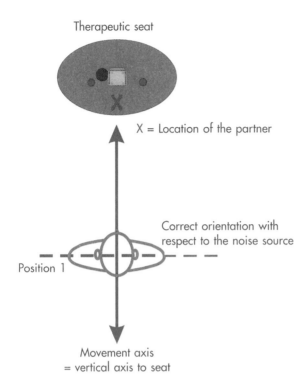

Therapeutic seat

X = Location of the partner

Correct orientation with
respect to the noise source

Position 1

Movement axis
= vertical axis to seat

In this diagram the listener is correctly oriented to the sound source, possibly after being adjusted by the partner.

Training Phase 1, Part 3

Follow these step-by-step instructions:

- Pause for about 20 seconds in this position, then move the listener on the front-back axis.

- Again, the partner takes secure but careful grasp of her shoulders. By gently pressing the listener backward and then forward by the shoulders, you will find the direction in which the next movement is performed. Choose the direction in which the listener moves most easily. If you are unsure which direction it is, lead her backward, farther from the therapeutic seat.

- The partner takes the listener in the chosen direction and then stops with her. Then the partner moves her upper body a few more times to the right and then to the left (gently, back and forth) to give her an opportunity to calmly juxtapose her feet and realign herself.

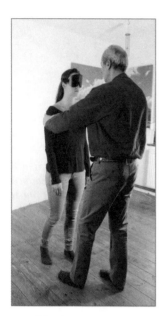

*Lead back, move together:
the partner presses lightly
on her shoulders in the
desired direction.*

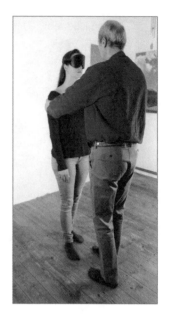

*Lead with
small steps.*

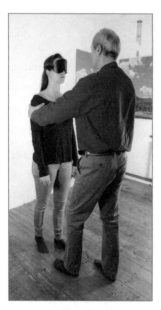

One more step . . .

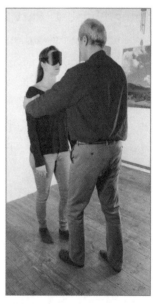

*Gently stop to allow her
feet to position themselves.*

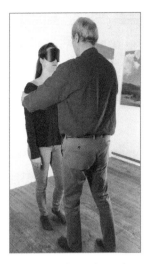 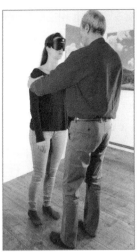 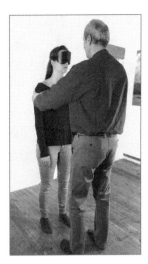

By applying lateral pressure in the direction of the movement, you give the listener an opportunity to juxtapose her feet.	*This lateral oscillating movement is smoothly executed so that she can also lift her other foot and align herself. This movement also relaxes the body.*	*After the oscillating adjustments, the listener is now correctly oriented in the direction of the sound source. Photos of this aspect of the exercise by Jutta Ebinger.*

- The partner returns to where the therapeutic seat is located and asks, "Where do you hear the singer? Please indicate with your hand, no matter where that is."
- The listener points to where she actually hears the singer's voice. This tells you how accurate her spatial orientation is.

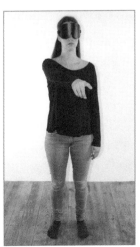

The person shows where in the room she hears the singer.

- This third part of the training phase is repeated several times until the listener hears the singer reasonably clearly from the front. At this point, with a strong hearing imbalance, it is sufficient that the singer is heard from the front area, but the singer's exact location need not be precise yet.

- To verify what has just taken place regarding the orientation to the music, the partner now serves as a second source of sound, asking, "Where do you hear me? Where am I? Please point, no matter where that is."

- The partner keeps asking this question until the listener has found the right direction and displays it by pointing at the partner. This location may be different from the position of the singer, or it may be the same position. This display makes it easier for you as the partner to develop a feel for how the correction process is progressing. As well, the listener can also determine how well the fine-tuning of her hearing sense is in terms of two sound sources.

- The partner's repeated question regarding his or her own position adds a second impulse to strengthen sound source orientation. The perception of the position of the partner is often more accurate than the perception of the singer because the partner is physically present and always in front of the listener, making actual physical contact with her. Thus the partner serves as a constant source of sound for the listener, unlike the singer, who is only a hologram in space and can be located only through pure auditory perception.

- This phase of the exercise may take some time. As the partner, always remember that this training is a very strenuous auditory exercise for the listener. If it takes longer and the positions are uncomfortable, take a short break or a moment of silence. Above all, the purpose here is to bring a sense of calm to the process and to avoid overloading the listener.

- Note: We always work with only songs 1 and 2. When the second song is over, go back to the first one. The maximum training time for this part of the exercise is approximately 20 minutes, which corresponds to the duration of both songs with one repetition. At this point you should stop and proceed to the debriefing.

Note to the Partner: Aligning Body Geometry

For the success of the basic method, it is crucial that the body geometry of the listener is properly aligned. This means that the head axis and/ or the shoulder axis are properly aligned, by the partner if necessary. Aligning means that the head and shoulder axes are parallel to each other and are perpendicular to the front-back axis.

As the partner, please be careful in making any adjustments to the alignment so that the listener doesn't get scared. To align the head, the partner uses both hands at the same time on both sides of the head, and to align the shoulders he uses both hands on the right and left upper arms of the listener, near her shoulders. As when moving the person in the room, you should always touch the listener gently, mindfully, and surely, and only align if a change is needed.

After the upper body, or shoulder axis, of the listener is aligned, you should then align the head. If the shoulders change while aligning the head—which is not unusual—then do not correct the shoulders afterward, as the body geometry is always determined by the head geometry.

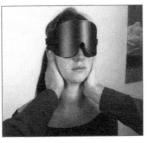

Adjust the head gently and mindfully.

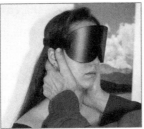

A lateral perspective of the hand position for the alignment of the head. Photos of this aspect of the exercise by Jutta Ebinger.

This intervention has a strong effect and must be carried out very sensitively, because any change to the usual posture can be very irritating to the listener. Correcting body geometry, especially the orientation of the head, is especially important when the position of the singer cannot be clearly identified and/or if the head position is wrong, as often happens with weak hearing. With weak hearing the listener will usually turn her head so that the stronger ear faces forward. However, in this position the head is no longer aligned with the sound source, making it hard to correct the difficulty in finding the location of the sound source.

If it's not possible to touch the listener (because she does not want to be touched or you don't want to touch her), the correction can also be done verbally. The partner says, for example: "Please turn your head slightly to the right" (or left, as the case may be). As you face the listener just remember that her right is your left, and vice versa. To adjust the height of the right shoulder, for example, say: "Please relax your right shoulder a bit." Try not to make more than 2 or 3 corrections in a training session of 20 minutes, because too many corrections can make the listener feel insecure.

To develop a well-balanced body geometry during the times between trainings, the listener will practice the mirror exercise from chapter 2 (pages 70 through 75) as part of their homework.

Training Phase 1, Part 4

Follow these step-by-step instructions:

- If and when the listener has clearly indicated that the singer is in front of her, an important milestone has been reached. The next step is for the listener to clearly hear the singer from the front but from different positions at least twice in a row. To do this, guide her to another position on the front-back axis and test this additional listening position according to the procedure from training phase 1, part 3.
- If part 4 of this training fails or the training phase takes too long (the total time of the training phase should be no more than

20 minutes), then you should stop this part of the training and try again after 1 to 3 days.

Pausing or Ending at Phase 1, Part 4

- Lower the music volume using the remote control until it is no longer audible, and then turn off the music. If you're already at the end of the second song, just let the music fade away. Then go to the listener and put a chair behind her so that the front edge of the chair touches the backs of her legs gently. Tell her that there is a chair behind her and ask her to sit down. Help her sit by securely holding her upper arms, as it may be that she feels somewhat uncertain during this process.
- Once the listener is seated, go over to the therapeutic seat, the one located in front of the sound equipment, and sit down facing the listener. Then say to her, "Please slowly take off the dark glasses."
- Ask her how she feels and what the experience was like for her. If a lot has happened, give her enough time to get back to normal.
- If the training is complete at this point, continue to "Downtime" (pages 178 through 179).

Note: When the Sound "Jumps"

In all stages of training it is possible that the perception of the position of the singer jumps sharply. For example, the listener hears the noise only from the side, then from the front, then possibly from behind. This can occur especially when a new position on the front-back axis is taken. This jumping phenomenon may also apply to the location of the partner's voice; however, this is more rare.

This sudden jump is a good sign, and the listener needs to be assured that this is so. It is a clear signal that the person has modified their usual hearing pattern and their system is looking for a new order. As I have said, in the beginning it's not important to be right, because with time and continued training the new order becomes set.

Training Phase 1, Part 5

Follow these step-by-step instructions:

- If the listener has clearly heard the singer from the front from two different positions on two consecutive occasions, then lead her to the therapeutic seat while the song is playing.

- Make sure that the starting position is not too far from the therapeutic seat because the "blind" walk in itself is a challenge. In this case, insert an intermediate station on the way to the therapeutic seat and ask the listener, "Where do you hear the singer? Where is the sound coming from? Please indicate with your hand, no matter where that is." As I said before, it's not about getting her to the seat quickly but about building a stable and well-established sense of space with the correct location of the sound source.

- When you reach the therapeutic seat, slowly turn the listener 180 degrees so that she is standing with her back to the seat. Ask the listener to sit down now, clasping her by her upper arms to support and stabilize her as she sits down.

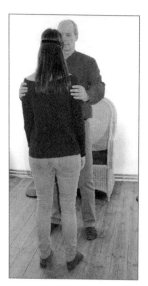 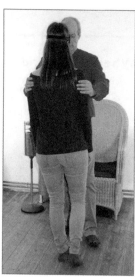 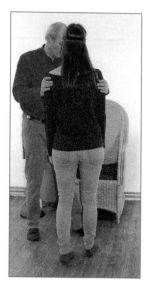

The partner holds the listener's upper arms to guide her to the seat.

The partner guides her to the seat.

Rotate (clockwise or counterclockwise) the listener in front of the seat.

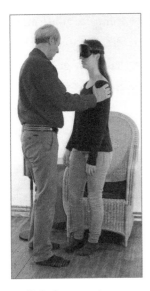

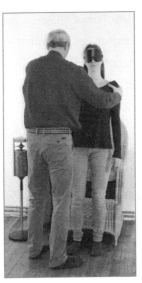

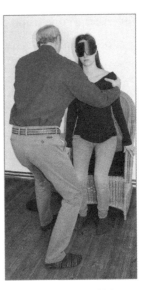

Help her turn in one smooth motion without releasing her shoulders.

Rotate her until she's in standing in front of the seat.

Continue to hold her shoulders as she sits down in the chair.

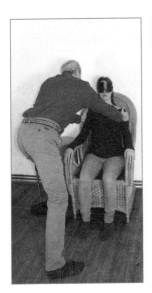

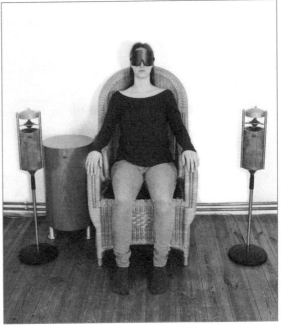

Help her to comfortably lean against the backrest of the seat. Photos of this aspect of the exercise by Jutta Ebinger.

The listener is now sitting relaxed in the seat and should hear the song directly behind her.

- At the conclusion of this part of the exercise, the complete adjustment of the auditory perception occurs (with the reference point at the back of the head, in accord with the fully balanced body geometry). The singing voice that has been heard from the front from different positions relative to the therapeutic seat is now clearly perceived from behind by the listener in the therapeutic seat. This creates a clear reference point for the acoustic perception in the listening field.

Training Phase 1, Part 6

Follow these step-by-step instructions:

- The music is usually perceived much louder seated within the hologram created by the Naturschallwandler natural sound transducer. Therefore you should set the volume slightly lower to start this part of the exercise.
- Let the listener, who is now sitting, hear the current musical piece, either song 1 or song 2, for a short time. Then turn the volume down gradually with the remote control until it is no longer heard, and then turn the music off completely.
- Sit down at a distance of about 2 yards from the listener in a chair, facing her.
- Tell her that she can remove the dark glasses or eyeshade and give her some time to return to herself.
- Please remain vigilant, monitoring and recording her reactions; for example, any changes in her complexion, expression, her mood, or whether she is relaxed.
- After you've turned off the music, ask the listener where she heard the sound coming from. After that, ask her how she feels and what her experience was like. At this point it is important that the listener shares everything that she feels at this moment.

Downtime

Before starting the final debriefing, give the listener a few moments to process her experience. This can be done in silence, or you could play the gentle sounds of the some meditative music or nature sounds such as flowing water or other peaceful and relaxing sounds. This supports the listener's stabilization and integration of the experience. If you use nature sounds, the volume should be as low as possible. As the partner, ensure a protected and undisturbed downtime. If a lot has happened, give the listener as much time as she needs.

Debriefing

Looking back, discuss the basic method in which a natural sound transducer such as the Naturschallwandler was used. What did the listener experience? What have you perceived as a partner? Be restrained and sensitive and allow the listener to reflect. As the partner in this process it makes sense to communicate to the listener your own observations regarding her movements and posture during the detection of the sound sources, including any changes in the volume of the music. In this way the listener is supported in perceiving how much her listening field moved and how she built this listening field herself.

Discuss the following:

- Results and observations of the training that has just been carried out.
- Additional actions.
- Schedule the next training dates.
- Exercises to do at home until the next training session to strengthen and further support the listening field; first and foremost for this kind of "homework" is the mirror exercise described in chapter 2 (pages 70 through 75). The remaining exercises, done at home, are described in the next chapters and are considered phase 2 of training.
- Clarify any questions.

It is important to emphasize to the listener that hearing improvement is based on continuous training. Arrange a training program consisting of 3 to 10 sessions to stabilize the hearing progress and to complete the overall process.

In phase 1, 2 appointments per week are ideal, with 1 to 2 days between appointments. Of course, the intervals between sessions can be longer, but not so long that what has been achieved is lost. That's why shorter intervals are recommended in the beginning—certainly no longer than 1 week. These can then be gradually extended over time.

If the perception of the location of the music or the partner's voice greatly moved during the exercise, it's important to explain that this is a very good sign that shows the body is seeking a new order.

Instructions to the Partner for Completing the Session

- What has changed in the listener's auditory perception, in their attitude, in their sense of volume, and so on?
- Note the spatial localizations of the listener if you have not already done so during the exercise.
- Please also read the "Conclusion to the Basic Method" below.

CONCLUSION TO THE BASIC METHOD

If you've followed this text so far, you might be unsure as to whether you have understood everything and done it right. That's why it's good to practice these step-by-step instructions with someone you know well—it does not have to be someone with a hearing deficit. Practice together. Practicing the basic method will strengthen your own hearing even if you don't have a hearing impairment.

I especially recommend that you, as the partner, experience the basic method from the perspective of the listener. This will clarify many questions you may have and allow you to discover firsthand how the method works, what is important, and what feels good.

The better you understand the basic principles of the method and gain personal experience from it, the more secure you will feel as a partner. As the sayings go, "There is no master who fell from the sky," and "Practice makes perfect!"

PART 1 ENDS—PART 2 BEGINS

You have now become familiar with the complete basic method and its various stages. Going through them all is the goal. Remember, it's not about getting it done as quickly as possible but about going through the various stages fully and completely.

The basic method is the foundation. On this foundation we can build and develop our hearing. Next, in part 2 of this book, we will look at the central aspects of the method in more detail and support them with additional elements, including exercises that can be done between sessions at home.

The Journey Is the Goal

Exercises that Further Support Hearing Regeneration

6

Being in the Present to Process the Past

Exercises to Find and Reflect
On the Triggering Event

THE THREE CENTRAL PILLARS

The three pillars of the method, *body geometry, spatial localization,* and *processing of perception,* are like keyboards that allow us to tap in to our system of perception and regulation. Concentrating on locating the sound source's location leads to an inner realignment and reorientation. If I align the body, feelings and related experiences are called forward. By opening up to images and sounds in my listening field I will automatically start to perceive them and relate them to my experiences. This makes the processing and evaluation of information clearer.

When we follow the steps in the exercises in the order in which they are given, we begin to change our inner programming to bring about improvement. Whether we have blocked and repressed certain traumatic aspects of our lives depends on how conscious we are of what happened. Processing always means understanding. Perhaps you remember a dispute that arose through a misunderstanding. The moment the misunderstanding is identified and clarified, the anger and pain largely dissolve. By remembering and understanding, blockages are processed, and new life opportunities develop.

The human body is a complex system of perception constructed according to certain proportions that are based on mathematical relationships that follow a given evolutionary order. This order is maintained by the 4 horizontal body axes and the vertical axis, which together stabilize the body and manifest its geometry. Through this body geometry, references for how we are oriented are created for 1) our inner perception (for example, position, posture, and balance) and 2) our external perception (for example, space, distance, height, movement, and speed). All the organs and functions of the body are aligned by this order and are involved in it. This also applies to our hearing. Through the body's geometry we communicate with our entire system, including the blockages and congestion that have manifested in the body. An important aspect here is our connection to the earth through the force of gravity. We touch the earth, and *the earth touches us.*

This spatial location gives us access to our individual library, in which all our experiences in relation to hearing are stored. Two factors are at play:

- Exterior factors: the accompanying impulses and the defined sound source
- Interior factors: a person's own work to align with the sound source

If the body cannot really adjust to the acoustic information it receives, stress is the result, as our system feels as though it is faced with something unknown. Through the use of a natural sound source or a natural sound transducer such as the Naturschallwandler, we can stimulate the ears and parts of the brain to relocate spatially so as to fully process the perceived sound information correctly.

In the course of training that includes working at different distances from the sound sources, in reality (through training and not by our imagination) we will sooner or later touch on traumatic experiences from the past that have resulted in hearing problems. Let's recall that trauma is always connected with space, in the sense that the traumatic situation, either physical or mental, affected my listening field such that it impaired my hearing. This was my feeling at the time of the trauma. It's not about blame; it simply means that because of this injury I hear worse. For the person concerned, this is reality, and we must always take another's reality seriously.

The partner always brings his own world into the process. Here a distinction is important: what I feel personally as a partner may be completely different from what the listener feels and is irrelevant to the training process itself. Training is not about coordinating the world of the partner and the listener but about creating a space of trust and perception in which the listener can recognize her own world without condemnation or blame. This, in conjunction with the strong desire to hear again, will—as surely as a magnet attracts a piece of iron—unveil the experiences stored by the listener that are associated with the hearing impairment. When there is unresolved trauma, it creates a burden. Initially the burden is always first felt and perceived because there is resistance. When there is no resistance, energy flows unimpeded through the entire body and the perception of sound is unclouded.

Passing through the rooms of my library of experiences, when I get in touch with a certain experience, it resonates with a burdensome memory that is now linked to my current situation. This may be in several ways: palpitations, nausea, sweating, strong movement of the sound source, and so on.

In training, this may happen when the sound source is perceived as deviating from the center axis, and after I change the distance to the sound source, this change in the reference point becomes a resonance point that sets off a memory of the original triggering event. Note that this resonance point is not static but moves—the sound source is perceived again and again from new directions in the listening field. This continues until we have largely digested the causal event. Then the locating—the accurate perception of the sound source—sets in naturally.

Perceptual space, like space in general, is always linked to geometry. The structure of space and thus each human body, the arrangement and mobility of its individual parts and proportions, determine how securely you move your body in space.

Pillar 1: Body Geometry and Divine Proportions

The divine origins of our body are found in its **proportions.** By perceiving our balance and symmetry through conscious movement like the exercises we do in our training method, we experience an internal order that promotes regulation.

> **Proportion:** The harmonious relation of parts to one another or to the whole; the relation of one part to another or to the whole with respect to magnitude, quantity, or degree (Latin, *proportio*, "symmetry")

The geometry of nature is reflected in the golden mean, also known as the golden ratio, in which the smaller portion (minor) to the larger (major) is always in the same proportion as the larger is to the whole. Its symbol is the Greek letter phi (Φ).

Minor	Major

├─────────────── The whole ───────────────┤

Minor : Major = Major : Whole
In figures = 1 : 1.6180339887. . . = Φ
The whole = 2.6180339887. . .

The formula for Phi is: $\Phi = \dfrac{\left(1+\sqrt{5}\right)}{2}$

It is of particular importance to our work that the golden ratio in humans is seen throughout the human body. In the human figure standing up, there is a ratio of 1 to 2, as seen in the sculpture of the figure on page 188. The proportions of each individual follow this rule. The upper body is proportionate to the lower body at a ratio of 1:2.

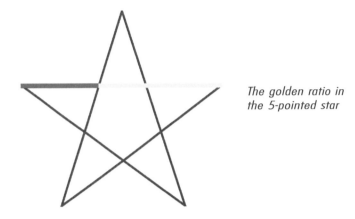

The golden ratio in the 5-pointed star

Respectively, the proportions of the upper body, as well as those of the lower body, also follow this rule.

Working on body geometry is important to restoring hearing because releasing trauma-induced blockages (tensions and twists) frees up stuck energy and restores the body to its correct proportions. For

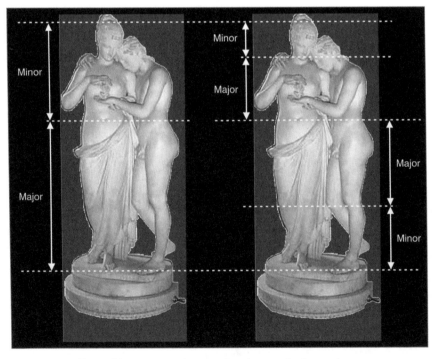

The golden ratio in the standing human body as shown in a jewelry-box sculpture

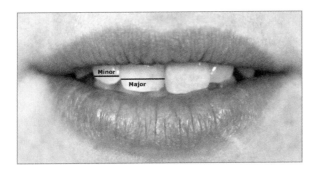

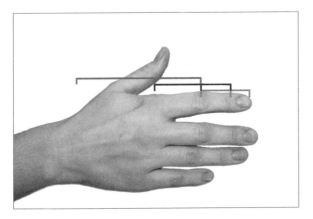

The golden ratio applies to each side of the body horizontally, as seen in the proportions of the teeth, fingertips, and limbs.

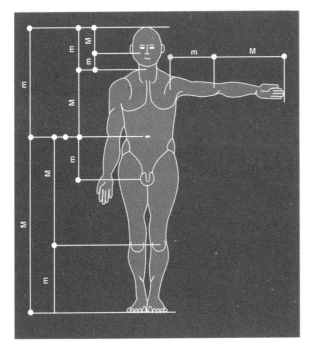

example, if an arm is broken or twisted, then the arm is proportionally no longer in its natural position due to the injury. If a part of the whole is off-center, the entire system will move from the middle because it must balance overall. The body reflects our experiences and adventures. Negative experiences always act in the direction of displacement of the natural order of the center. An imbalance in the body automatically creates additional tension and therefore more force is needed to keep this shift from moving away from the center. An example: We sprain our foot and try to relieve this by placing more weight on the other, uninjured, side. This naturally makes us compensate for the imbalance as the sprained foot heals. However, if the healing (self-regulation) of the sprained foot is not complete, a degree of imbalance remains. We must now consciously regulate this imbalance if we want to regenerate the injured foot completely.

Sometimes it's necessary to give the body an impulse that allows it to get back to its natural balance. For example, if we've broken a bone, we stabilize the fracture into its correct position as it was before the break by splinting or putting the appendage in a cast. This solid stability gives the body the impulse it needs to regulate and heal. We do the same thing for the body when restoring hearing. Repeatedly aligning the body geometry as we do in the training exercises gives the body a sense of safety and orientation. True, the process of repeating these exercises can sometimes seem monotonous while we're building a new pattern in the body. However, the consistency of this repetition helps create the stability that promotes the body's self-regulation.

Pillar 2: Spatial Localization

Spatial orientation is just as important as hearing itself. Both are processed in tandem by our brain with every sound we perceive. Spatial orientation is a critical element of hearing. Often we notice that we understand everything well in a quiet room, but as soon as we walk into a space with ambient noise, such as a car, we have difficulty understanding others. This happens because we don't have a good location—we're not usually aware that this is the case, and instead we think we're hearing poorly due to our advancing age.

In a one-on-one conversation I can relatively easily correct my positioning with my eyes. I do this subconsciously and automatically: I know that when the other person is speaking, the sound of his words must be coming from where he is. All this comes together in my brain, which calculates the sound and the location of the source of the sound. This assignment of sounds is the function of the hearing sense and of one's spatial orientation. If I need my eyes to locate the source of a sound, this slows down the perceptual process and increases the amount of energy required to hear. And this can put me under stress, which is why I tire more quickly in situations where it's hard to hear.

If additional ambient sounds are added to the mix, these too are immediately located by my brain. After all, I always hear my entire environment and must then decide which sounds I want to focus on while ignoring extraneous sounds. However, if the location is not completely intact—that is, if a sound and its allocation in space do not coincide precisely—my brain will immediately become overloaded. I can correct one incorrect location by using my eyes, but several locations of simultaneously perceived noises are much more difficult to correct since my brain can only correct one error at a time. That's why I need the other person to speak louder so that this source is separated from the background noise and can be perceived by me. And so if I have a hearing impairment, I will always have a difficult time locating the source of sound, and I have to look in order to hear: "Ah, it's because someone just spoke," or "Oh, there's the car."

Spatial localization begins almost at birth. Gradually we assign sounds to things: That is Mom when she's happy. That's Mom when she's angry. That's Dad. That is a car. That is the dog. That is my brother and sister. That is a thunderstorm. That clatter means soon we will eat—and many, many more sounds.

We learn in the classroom of life what individual sounds mean. Normally we grow better in this learning process; we learn to assign more precisely, to link words and understand relationships. But as we have seen, there are times in life as a result of traumatic experiences when the opposite process prevails, and we unlearn. And here begins many hearing impairments. The aim of our work is to come back to a natural way of hearing in which the identification and perception of sound comes naturally and properly and is connected to its spatial allocation.

There are animals who have perfected spatial localization: bats, whales, and dolphins, for example. These beings have a very highly evolved sound-based localization system that includes ultrasound. If the acoustic detection of a bat is disturbed in the slightest, then it is lost, it can no longer catch mosquitoes, and it's in danger of hitting a wall in the dark or colliding with other bats.

A 2014 German radio broadcast reported on Israeli researchers who had discovered special neurons in rat and mouse brains that serve as two-dimensional directional signs. Neurobiologist Arseny Finkelstein commented, "What surprised me was just how similar rats and bats are. In evolution, they have been separated for millions of years. They also show very different behavior. Yet they have neurons with similar functions in the same brain regions. This means that this sense of direction of the evolutionary mechanism is very old. Therefore, we think that there ought to be something very similar in humans, as well."[1]

Many hearing-impaired persons cannot filter out background noise when it comes to isolating and focusing on a specific sound source, such as a conversation partner. This is a frequent problem, particularly for hearing aid users. The auditory environment becomes one large canvas of noise in which the pieces of information can no longer be distinguished from the background. All sounds together become undefined noise.

This can be significantly improved and corrected by training in the basic therapeutic method presented in this book. A prerequisite for the optimization of perception is to first establish a clearly defined listening axis. We learn where the front is and where the back is. This basic mapping that we may regard as banal is not so obvious in reality. This is why people sometimes say, "You don't know your front from your rear!" We hear a noise and can't tell exactly where it's coming from without training. If the listening axis is not established, there's resistance against order. That's not wrong; it's just important that we know there is a resistance.

Pillar 3: The Processing of Perception

Our perceptual system must map the world for us to understand it and find our way around in it. A sound event is always a challenge that is received by our body. In the brain, this acoustic sensory stimulus

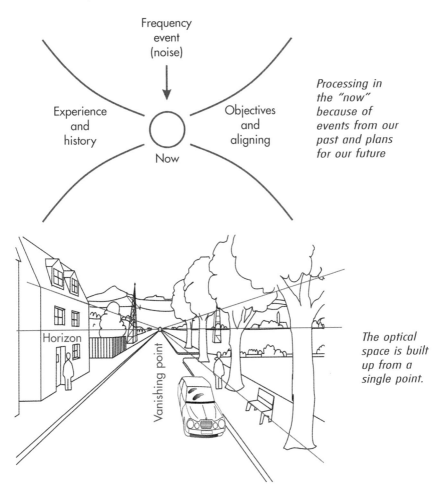

Frequency event (noise)

Experience and history

Objectives and aligning

Now

Processing in the "now" because of events from our past and plans for our future

Horizon

Vanishing point

The optical space is built up from a single point.

immediately calls forth a neural response from hidden (unconscious or subconscious) and open (conscious) knowledge. We respond in the here and now always with the experience and knowledge of our history and our current orientation, which is determined by our goals and intentions for the future. The processing of perception is a very complex pillar of the basic method because it involves many aspects.

We need two eyes to see spatially and to look into the depths of space. Also, the optical space is from one point (the vanishing point): it is where all perspective lines converge.

With only one eye we see increasingly flat and two-dimensional. This is also true for the ears: with two healthy ears we hear spatially in all directions; with only one ear, listening flattens out and makes for a confusion in orientation. You can easily check this for yourself by keeping one eye or one ear closed off for a few minutes. The displacement and confusion of perception is quickly felt.

Every moment of hearing, whether it is a bird singing or a voice raised in anger, always involves locating and classifying, a process in which my entire system automatically takes an active part. I can only perceive with the participation of all of my senses. Most of the time this happens subconsciously. Perception therefore means processing, mapping, and evaluating with all my senses.

EXERCISE: Perceiving a Sound with All the Senses

Follow these step-by-step instructions:

Close your eyes and listen for the first sound that you can hear.

- How does it feel? Where do you feel it in the body, especially?
- What does this sound taste like?
- What does this sound look like in your mind?
- How does the sound smell?
- Finally, how did you hear the sound? Is it loud or quiet? Does it sound good? What other sense reacts?

Comments and hints: The point of this exercise is to become more aware of the complex perception of sound. Above all, if we want to process traumatic aspects, it may be helpful to visualize not only the audio impressions but also the other stored sensory impressions so that those stressful events that are still alive in us today yet dormant can be perceived and processed.

The preceding exercise is associated with understanding and self-knowledge: How do I experience something? How do I feel something? Do I like it or don't I like it? Do I find it beautiful or not? Am I happy or not? To clarify this for yourself has a liberating effect. An elderly woman told me in a lengthy interview that ever since she trained with the basic method she's processed many old war events. She said that it was easy for her. She experienced images and dreams as a result of the training but was able to just let them pass through, and now she feels liberated from the trauma of those past events. This is a form of self-knowledge. She had not felt like this for years, she told me, so light and relaxed.

With training one tends to accept events just as they are. Without doing so one continues to feel stuck. With training, emotions like anger, rage, and disappointment weigh less and less, and we feel less oppressed. The past was as it was, and the more I understand the past, the easier it is for me to be in the here and now. By building order in my listening field by resolving old traumas and tensions, I find it easier and easier to just be present and let go of events of the past.

And since unprocessed stressful events also affect me physically, I can work through many types of physical problems by emotionally and mentally processing past traumas. Many therapeutic approaches show that the body is a way to access and connect with consciousness. The body and consciousness work in conjunction.

We all want to feel good in our bodies. When I'm sick or have pain or severely impaired function, it's no longer easy for me to feel good. I may be able to live with it, but it would be so much nicer if my body, with all its functions, would stay healthy. We have the power of the mind to compensate for pain and limitations and still be happy, but if we can eliminate all or some of this pain, our quality of life is enhanced, and new body dynamics and renewed strength will support a much more constructive, optimistic way of thinking.

TENSION AND BALANCE

Tension plays a very important role in the human body. To be able to walk upright and move, we have to build a certain amount of tension in the body. This is achieved by our muscles, tendons, ligaments, and connective tissue. The control of these processes is done through the voluntary nervous system. The involuntary nervous system is responsible for controlling the processes that occur without our conscious intervention, such as the heartbeat or bowel movements.

Decisive in this tension is the balance of the entire system; otherwise it becomes unbalanced. If we have too much tension somewhere in the body and too little tension in another location, the body twists, stretches, or bends in specific areas or even overall.

In particular, fine motor control (such as taking a step) requires precise balancing and alignment. Our state of tension—whether it is in balance or out of balance—determines whether our movements are fluid and elegant or clumsy and awkward. This is not a matter of aesthetics—it is about whether the body is without stress and thus, being in balance, can maintain its functions as it ages.

The following exercise is an exploration of how the body uses tension to maintain balance.

((•)) EXERCISE: Walking Straight Ahead

Follow these step-by-step instructions:
- First, take a few steps forward as you usually walk.
- Then, consciously straighten and tighten the body's posture and breathe 2 or 3 times in and out deeply.

- Now, slowly and with great control, take a few steps again.
- Repeat the sequence from the beginning.
- Is there a difference between the first way of walking and second way? Feel the difference?
- How does your body feel now?

Comments and hints: By slowly walking, we strengthen the control of our body. Weak or not, precise hearing is also, in a way, a function of muscular control of the body. Inner ear bones are held in place through muscular alignment.

All movements of the muscles are controlled by the brain. Through the practice of consciously slowly walking, I can strengthen my control. Since all processes in the body are connected, I can perceive other movements more consciously by paying attention to the complex process of walking. Similarly, by listening more consciously and more deliberately, I can improve the fine muscular control of my hearing process. Another benefit of this controlled walking exercise is that I can train myself to become more conscious of the alignment of my body and thus move more precisely in my space. Therefore my body feels safer in the way it moves through space.

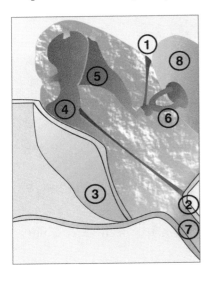

Inner ear bones are held in place and aligned by muscles and tendons. These are the hammer (4), the anvil (5), and the stirrup (6), which connect the eardrum (3) with the cochlea (8). They bridge the interior of the middle ear, which merges with the Eustachian tube (7). The tension and suspension of these three tiny inner ear bones happens via three tendonlike ribbons (blue in the sketch) and two small muscles (red in the sketch). The stapedius (1) sits at the foot of the stirrup and is innervated (stimulated and controlled) by a side branch of the facial nerve, the nerve stapedius. The tensor tympani (2) comes in at the bottom of the hammer, ranging on the opposite side, where it ends at the beginning of the Eustachian tube. Innervation is via the vagus tensor tympani, a side branch of the mandibular nerve.

When we stand balanced and in our center, we have the same basic tension in all the major muscles, as well as a smooth and balanced flow of energy.

If the tension in the body is very different in one part of the body than in another, I'll have problems with movement. The energy is not flowing properly, and we sometimes feel this as pain. If the transitions between movements are not smooth, there will be congestion or weakness. And if the tension in one part of the body is too different from another part of the body, it is hard to achieve balance in our system.

By building our sense of balance, our energy levels balance out, and thus our entire energy flow becomes more fluid. That's why people in training usually increase the body's temperature, even to the point of starting to sweat, while only making physically small movements.

The following exercise is designed to explore our sense of balance.

EXERCISE: Balance and Control

This exercise is done with a partner. Follow these step-by-step instructions:

- Stand (or sit if standing is not possible) face-to-face with your partner.
- The partner points to an arm or a leg on your body.
- First, imagine how you move this part of your body. Only when you feel completely safe and ready, perform the movement.
- Now lift your arm or leg and then bring it back to the starting position.
- If the you can perform this exercise without any problems, then you can increase the difficulty level by having your partner give you a verbal command rather than pointing to the body part; for example, "Lift your left leg."
- Continue with commands and corresponding actions for about 5 minutes.
- Always end the exercise after a movement has been carried out correctly.

Comments and hints: In this exercise, as with all others, precision is important, not speed. We are trying to bring thought and intention together with physical implementation, even if it is incomplete or shaky. If the trainee first thinks until they're sure which part of the body should be moved, and then performs the movement, this will strengthen the control of the body and build a sense of security.

IF YOU BELIEVE IT, YOU WILL SEE IT!

You have already read a lot of information on regulation, effects, and how to improve your sense of hearing. You have learned, trained, and done the exercises. The order of the exercises given in this book is a process that addresses your total system from various angles, and, most important, gives you a sense of what regulation means and how it works. You might have already experienced some positive changes. If not, you may be questioning whether this system works. Are you asking yourself: *Is this really true? Does this all make sense? Can my hearing really improve?*

Something is only useful for us if it matches the way we structure our consciousness. Consciousness is structured by the assumptions we make, the beliefs we adopt, and the decisions we make. One idea might be fantastic, clever, and meaningful for one person, yet completely ridiculous to another.

It's quite natural to question, and I tell you straight away, do not believe anything without checking it out first. Nevertheless, for you to truly verify something as true, you must first accept at least the *possibility* that it works; otherwise you won't get anywhere.

I cannot resolve this question for you. Listen to your inner voice to decide whether you will keep training.

People say, "I'll believe it when I see it." My response is, "No, if you believe it, *then* you'll see it." You can see it because your belief in the possibility creates a reality.

Faith means we open ourselves up to a possibility and know that our aspirations *can* become reality, even when we don't know when and how.

To be therapeutically successful, I must base my method of restoring hearing on natural law. Laws of nature have determined our evolution from the beginning. We have a clear sense of this, and we know intuitively whether something is in accord with natural law. On this basis we are constantly reviewing all our new impressions. Our consciousness perceives the outcome of this review in the form of our feelings.

Whether a project or a goal seems real or achievable depends on how we feel about it. If we feel good about it, even when we don't know *how* it can be realized, it gives us the motivation to open to the possibility and take steps toward achieving the goal without feeling any pressure or demand. If we do not feel good about it, we can change the goal until we do feel good about it. If we see no possibility, it makes no sense to pursue the goal—we would only confirm what we already know: that we cannot achieve it.

RESOLVING TRAUMA

To work on trauma, whether physical or mental, we have to understand the circumstances of its beginning as clearly and precisely as possible. It is critical to find the starting point of the trauma, because the triggering worked like an input program and changed our whole system on the mental, physical, and emotional levels. In particular, it created chronically higher stress levels within the system.

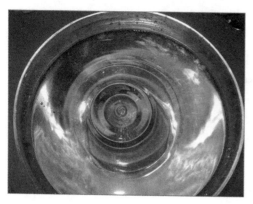

Trauma is like a strike. In this image, a single drop of water strikes a full glass. Just as a single drop of water can change the order of a system, trauma can have a similar impact on the human system.

Normally this input program, once it has served its purpose—to control, for example, the healing of a tympanic membrane injury—is replaced by the basic program for the return of control—that is, the normal state—and the organ concerned would work again according to its specific function. Any resulting limitations due to scarring would be largely compensated for by our overall system so that we would hardly notice a weakening in everyday life.

However, when the normal program does not turn on after physical healing is complete, it's because parts of the traumatic event were displaced due to excessive pain, and therefore these parts could not be fully processed. The original event and the related effects are then partially obscured and not fully accessible by our conscious mind. Thus the trauma program remains active, constantly running in the background. It's important to remember that trauma is processed by both the body and the soul according to a universal order, but felt and experienced in very individual ways.

Once we recognize order—which is why it is so important to do so—we have the opportunity, even the responsibility, and to act in accordance with this recognized order. I can only act and control in a system that is subject to order. A chaotic system, then, can only be changed by a considerable expenditure of energy and only in isolated areas, but without profound and lasting stability.

Targeted effort and natural forces can regulate a system with an underlying order, but I can only regulate this order if I have experienced this order and my mind understands it. This order is expressed, for example, in various phases, as shown in the schematic diagram of a wave. Without a complete cycle, without an up phase and a down phase, there cannot be a complete wave and the next wave cannot form. There is no tomorrow without the evening.

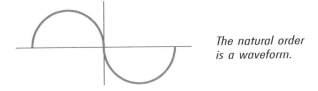

The natural order is a waveform.

Each child tries to develop a certain order in his or her bedroom (although it often doesn't look like that to outsiders). They do this because order is a basic principle of life. Order is in fact half of life—the other half being the person's development of this order. All people try to create a lasting order to navigate their world. But events such as trauma can make the basic order rigid, fixed, and immutable. Natural rhythms and the inherent ability to self-heal and self-regulate are affected. For example, an ability such as hearing doesn't come back, or a ringing sound (tinnitus) remains.

We are always causally involved in a traumatic event. If this weren't so, there would be no way to heal. In the basic method of regenerating hearing, we see that we ourselves have set up our listening field and therefore we ourselves can organize it and change it. Theodor Schwenk said:

> There can be in one place only *one* solid body but *many* and diverse movements. This is an important universal principle; structures are imposed upon space, arranging and dividing it up according to systematic laws. This shows movement to be independent of space, though *appearing* in it as a regulating principle (emphases in original).[2]

The 3 biological factors that are part of a trauma—shock, isolation, and dramatic significance—cause a button to be pressed. The computer that is our biology will then start a whole new program. Our task is to resolve the emotional conflict caused by the traumatic experience so that on the physical level our system can return to its regular function and normal order. If we succeed in our goal we will come to a new understanding. That's what we see so wonderfully in every child who gets sick and then recovers: once they've gone through the illness and the healing process, they're stronger, clearer, and have grown as a result of it. Although they may still be a bit physically weak, they have undergone an evolution.

Let's now consider some practical exercises to help us find the traumatic experience underlying a condition such as hearing loss.

(((•)) Finding the Triggering Event

The more I accurately and completely recall the situation that triggered my weakness or my physical symptoms, the sooner I can find a solution to the conflict that underlies it. To this end, following are some questions to ask yourself.

What is my current situation?
Beginning on the physical level:
- What has changed physically? What happens in my body, exactly?
- What is the correct medical diagnosis?

Next, on the intellectual and spiritual level:
- What is the problem?
- What is the pain?
- When does the pain occur?

How does this situation affect my life?
- What am I not able to do anymore?
- What should I not do because of my physical condition?
- Do I behave differently? (For example, with hyperacusis, I need to withdraw.)
- How does it feel? How does it affect my life? Do I not hear certain sounds, or are they strengthened? Do I not hear well only in certain situations? Can I no longer understand individuals well?

Since when have I had this condition?
- When did it start?
- What exactly happened?
- What were the circumstances surrounding the event?
- How did I feel then as I experienced the situation?

Note: It is important that we remember this triggering event that has caused our system to weaken. Is there always such an originating traumatic event? Yes! Although we are not always aware of a particular incident, there must be one. It's like looking at your body and discovering a scar—your hearing loss. This is the causal underlying event, the concrete realization of any trauma.

Where is this going? What do I want?

Without clear knowledge of what caused your current physical and spiritual reality, you cannot change purposefully. If you are "in the clouds" with regard to the cause of your current state, you have no ground on which you can stand.

When asked what we want, the task is to formulate a goal positively, saying, "What do I *really* want? What is my direction?" We don't want to frame this as a negative, as in "I don't want this or that anymore." The topic "Clear Goals" is covered in chapter 10.

In the next chapter, we first take a look at the perception of inner and outer space.

7

I Hear, Therefore I Am
Exercises to Recover Orientation

WE LIVE IN A THREE-DIMENSIONAL WORLD that we share with all other beings. Everything in this space constantly vibrates, each particle, each being. Each being's vibration is perceived by all other beings and is an expression of the energy of the collective field of energy.

Sound is one of these vibrations. Light is vibration too, but in such a high frequency that we cannot hear it. The elements of sound, its frequency and vibration, are its tones, which are expressive of a mood or an emotion. The German word *Ton* (sound) flipped around is *Not* (distress). You could say that sound is a necessity. A spontaneously performed song helps us alleviate suffering. Most likely we have each sung or listened to a song to help us feel more courageous. Singing and whistling signal to my surroundings, "I'm here, and this is my territory." In this way, sound can mark a boundary.

Countless legends and fairy tales from different cultures and eras tell how witches, magicians, and sorcerers conjured up something by means of mostly rhythmically spoken words, causing a transformation of matter. Speech is syllable-shaped sound and has the potential to form and transform matter. In fact, talking is always a design and creation process. Words have power; they can hurt, and they can heal.

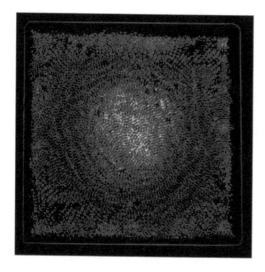

Water sound image of Tibetan monks chanting. Vibration is always an expression of power and a certain quality. Photo by Alexander Lauterwasser from his book Wasser, Klang, Bilder *(AT Verlag: Aarau, 2002).*

We connect with the holographic nature of the world by means of vibrations. This is the subject of this chapter.

HOLOGRAMS CONNECT AND RESONATE WITH THE WORLD

When we hear, we strive to create the most complete picture of the external world within us. In other words, we create a hologram of the entire world, with all its oscillations and complex information, within ourselves.

As noted earlier, the word *hologram* is made up of two Greek words, *holos*, "whole, complete," and *gramma*, "weight, letter, written." Even the smallest part of a hologram contains all the information of the whole. At the same time, the hologram is special in that it allows us to have a spiritual experience at any time: an experience of profound happiness, an experience of understanding, a special contact with another person, a connection to an animal—there are countless possibilities to experience.

If we go to a special place, a powerful sacred space, our holographic ability to communicate with the world around us is enhanced. When we are connected to our environment, especially with the beings we love, it is easier for us to deepen and align our own perceptions.

A good friend of mine has created such a place of power in nature, a seat near his house that he goes to regularly to meditate, contemplate, or simply to sit in silence. It can be very supportive to have such a place. Such a special place may even be in one's own home.

When we observe nature, we always find order and structure. It pervades the entire universe, from the smallest atomic particle to the largest galaxy. Even rational scientists are often amazed at the beauty and precision of the orderly phenomena of nature.

Nature's inherent order is also reflected in our individual organisms. Nature does not do anything "just like that"; it follows an order. The more I come to understand that the principles of nature apply to me, the better I can understand what is happening within me.

For instance, if I lose my bearings, it becomes difficult to act sensibly. If I get lost in the woods, it makes little sense to go in any direction without first trying to orient myself. Or consider a small child who has lost his mother and goes into a panic. That's exactly what we experience as adults when we lose our orientation. We probably don't start to scream and howl like a young child, but the inner feelings of being lost have a similar energy and trigger a similar fear. These are basic biological principles that manifest in a parallel fashion on the soul level. Even if I initially reject something or am afraid of it, it is nevertheless a part of me that wants to be perceived and understood.

The recovery of one's orientation is one of the reasons why we emphasize relaxation while doing the exercises that comprise the basic therapeutic method. This helps us create (or re-create) an orderly interior space. With that, the following exercise is offered.

EXERCISE: Blindfolded Identification of Sounds and Their Location

Follow the instructions below:

- Set aside 10 minutes to 1 hour to do this exercise—as long as this exercise is fun and stimulating. If possible, do this exercise outdoors. You will be describing noise while blindfolded and show-ing a partner where the sound is coming from by pointing. The following are examples, but the concept applies to all sounds that are just perceptible.

- ▸ What kind of car do I hear? (Is it a truck, bus, or small or big car?)
- ▸ Where is this car, and is it moving?
- ▸ Where is the bird whose chirping I hear?

- The partner provides feedback as to whether the direction shown is correct. If it's not correct, the partner describes where the noise source is; for example, more to the right, more to the left, higher, lower, and so on. You will try again to find the correct location by pointing until your partner confirms that you're right. The partner may need to correct the placement by hand until it is correct.

- This exercise can be done in a group or as a fun exercise with chil-dren. One person serves as the partner while all the others are blindfolded (or close their eyes). If you are the partner, you can describe a perceptible noise and ask the participants to show by hand where they hear the sound and then open their eyes to check their accuracy.

Comments and hints: The idea behind this exercise is to identify all the different sounds that can be heard in your listening field. Distinguish louder and quieter sounds, melodic sounds like the song of a bird, and complex sounds such as the rustling of leaves.

REGAINING VITALITY

In January 2017, a woman called me who had recovered her spatial orientation by training in the method. She said, "I now have a new motto: 'I listen, therefore I am.'" After she made tremendous prog-ress with her hearing, new worlds opened up for her. She told me that she had returned many times to a time in her childhood during

World War II that she once had a hard time accessing. She only realized this now since she can hear much better. As a result, she has a new, more positive attitude toward life. For a long time she had many, sometimes terrible, dreams of her early life during the war, and now she clearly realizes how much those traumas shaped her experience of the past and her present. "Only now that I hear again do I realize what I have missed," she said.

Painful experiences shape us. Sometimes we build a protective shield that will not let us feel so much. Outwardly we seem to be somewhat cold and stiff, while inwardly we feel cut off. Once we are able to recall these old experiences and traumas and reestablish our internal order, we can regain our vitality and in the process better understand ourselves.

Let us deepen our understanding of the restoration of control and order in the chapter that follows.

8
Each Ship Has a Helmsman
*Exercises to Take Control
and Restore Order*

IN DAILY LIFE, THE CONTROL AND POSITIONING of our system, our internal order and the assignment of all sounds according to this order, act automatically as an interconnected occurrence within us. We had to learn order once, and this was a natural process. The more we learned, the more this process became automatic. We were able to compensate for minor deviations in our established internal order, but at some point we realized, *Oh, I don't hear so well anymore.* Here is where it's possible to consciously rebuild our internal order, starting with stabilizing and aligning our body geometry. Recall the vertical and horizontal axes that stabilize and manifest the geometry of the body.

Every living being has an internal order, a control system. For human beings, this is centered on the physical level primarily in our brain and nervous system as well as in the structure of the body. It's what gives us both uniformity and diversity. We can easily tell by looking at our fellow human beings that despite each person's unique form, we are all the same in our basic structure (two eyes, two ears, organs, muscles and bones, tissues, cells, etc.).

If we properly address our common control system at a fundamental level, it will lead us back to our original order. We will be delving into this subject in the following chapters. The exercises here are intended to strengthen this self-regulation process.

THE BRAIN, OUR HOLOGRAPHIC HUB

The brain is a holographic element where the central aspects of our being are located. We specifically recognize three aspects:

- It is physically present as an organ in our body.
- It has aspects such as memory functions and possibilities of perception that we cannot locate on the organic level of the brain.
- It's a control center for our consciousness.

On the physical level, the brain controls all our bodily functions, from processes that restore our internal order when we are sick or injured, to sophisticated procedures that have developed over millions of years in our collective evolution. From brain research we know that memory and intelligence are functions that cannot really be localized, that these are holographic: in each part, the whole is represented and functionally designed. Neurobiologist Gerald Hüther reports that a man who had a very small brain nevertheless led a normal life.[1] This example and many others of people who retained almost complete brain function after a brain injury shows us that our thinking organ always works as a whole in a way that is not completely understood. Apparently the brain can compensate for component failures. On the other hand, there are examples in which relatively small regions or parts of the brain have been injured or damaged—for instance, by stroke—yet lead to severe disability and limitation of physical and mental abilities.

Scientific research shows that consciousness is indeed coupled with our physical body, and yet is not part of our physical system. Near-death experiences; spiritual phenomena such as clairvoyance or spontaneous healing; specific physical abilities of monks and yogis, especially in the Far East; the mental and physical feats of martial artists and professional athletes—all these have one thing in common: our consciousness governs and controls matter. The physical body, the control center that is the brain and our consciousness, is engaged in a constant exchange of information and feedback from within and without.

The following is an exercise in controlled consciousness.

EXERCISE: Get Up and Sit Down

Follow these step-by-step instructions:
- Begin in the seated position, stand briefly, then sit down again.
- Now visualize yourself repeating this exercise. Imagine in your mind how you would perform the exercise.
- Now stand again, rest briefly, then sit down again.
- This exercise can also be done in reverse. Begin in the standing position, sit down, then stand up again.

Comments and hints: Your consciousness has formulated a will to execute this action that has gone from your brain to your body. Did you find the movement easier after visualizing it first? Did it feel different? Was the movement the second time more fluid? Was it implemented with less effort? We use this same exchange of information when it comes to releasing blockages in our listening system.

OUR BODY STORES ALL OUR EXPERIENCES

Traumatic experiences always manifest on a physical level in the form of blockages or a reduction of functionality. For recovery we need awareness of the traumatic event, because awareness is our helmsman, so to speak; "he" needs to realize what happened and process the stressful situation to recover our natural internal order. Only then can "he" chart a new course.

By working with the body, we interact with our consciousness and get feedback. In the basic method, by addressing the body through the three pillars (body geometry, spatial localization, and the processing of perception), past experiences are called up, as if we were clicking on an image on the computer that now becomes visible. In this way we can experience and consciously process our feelings in the here and now, reevaluating the traumatic experience so that we can return to our natural order. Again, I point this out because it is important that we understand the processes involved in restoration and do not think we can solve anything by working with the physical body alone without addressing the underlying trauma. Awareness is always crucial to this process.

If we are very tense and do stretching exercises, tension decreases. This is good. The support and care of the body, especially if we are physically ill or our bodily functions need strengthening, is important. This is where medicine has achieved outstanding results. But as long as the underlying issue is not resolved, what is actually behind the physical symptoms will eventually lead to the body becoming tense again.

I cannot process trauma that has led to my constant neck pain by doing a relaxing exercise that only focuses on the physical symptoms, but by making myself conscious of the underlying trauma and then doing the physical exercise, I can access my deeper emotions underlying the pain. I can call up the associated emotions from my subconscious and bring them back into my consciousness to begin the process of healing. It is often possible to partially process traumatic events by facing the trauma in the here and now. All of a sudden I realize, "Oh, I feel stronger. I am able to stand up straight, and nobody will intimidate me today!"

Recovering Hearing in the Left Ear

Mrs. H. after an intensive training said, "It is as if the new orientation can heal an old blockage or an injury. That is why I want to repeat this exercise as often as possible to deepen my success.

"For this wonderful listening experience I am deeply grateful. In retrospect, I came to my hearing loss in my left ear from a theme that was persistent in my early childhood, which was 'I do not know where I belong.' You said at the final meeting that behind every manifestation of complaints, a theme is hidden. This realization can be much help in efforts to cure us."

Sometimes we can't avoid the storms of life, the traumas. They happen to nearly all of us. Although we keep looking forward, those past experiences belong to our existence: sometimes they manifest in ways we do not want to experience. Traumatic experiences that settle in the body always proceed according to clear structures and patterns, but at the same time they also give us clues as to how they can be resolved. We address these healing processes in the next section.

THE BRAIN AS CONTROL CENTER

If a painful experience surprises me and I feel alone and abandoned, then the three factors—*shock, isolation,* and *dramatic significance*—come together to create a traumatic crisis situation in which I feel so threatened that I cannot think straight. This is the activation of a survival program. The brain stem, which is the transition region between the spinal cord and the brain itself, takes the lead when the other brain functions are confused. In particular, the cerebrum, which is normally responsible for rational decisions and solutions as well as the movement of the body, is in a state of shock in the case of severe traumatic situations, causing us to freeze.

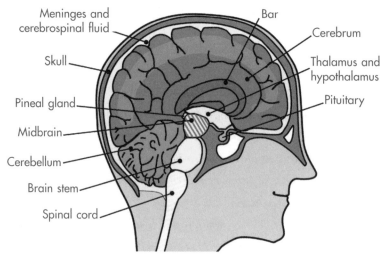

A lateral view of the brain

The repertoire of the brain stem consists of three programs: fight, flight, and if the first two are not possible, paralysis. For example, if I have a relationship with someone but I have a serious conflict in which I would not attack or run away from that person—for example, I have a dispute with my boss, whom I cannot attack because I might get fired—I have a situation in which neither fight nor flight are options. In this case the third program comes into play: I freeze and am unable to do anything at all. To resolve this situation I need to move. This is how our basic method works as well. We find that through movement we can resolve the deadlocked situation through a series of step-by-step movements that allow the cerebrum to regain control. Only our consciousness may ultimately find the solution for the healing of a traumatic situation.

Traumatic events are always associated with stress. This places excessive demands on the system, causing the two halves of the brain to vibrate differently. When that happens, the whole system becomes unbalanced because we feel divided and unable to work as a unified whole. The combination of emotion and rationality breaks apart. We are then dominated by one side of the brain or the other. We either ignore our feelings, or we become overwhelmed by our feelings and cannot think straight, so we just react.

The cranial nerves originate in the brain stem. The brain stem is directly involved in the management of our neurological system and is concerned with basic survival (it regulates our heartbeat and digestive system, for instance) and is not subject to our will or consciousness. It controls stress and relaxation, from a fast heartbeat to fatigue after a long, hard day. The brain stem does not differentiate between the hemispheres; it operates as a single unit. It works along the lines of in/out. Accordingly, it controls our food intake, digestion, and elimination, as well as heartbeat and bowel movements. There is no left-right principle here, that only begins in the midbrain.

Therefore the forward and backward movements that we use in the basic method act on the brain stem and midbrain. The simple act of moving forward to the sound source or away from it has a physiological effect on the brain stem that is relaxing. And through this, the areas of the brain that follow in the chain of events get a chance to take hold and to plug into the action again.

These movements, especially when performed barefoot, have an especially relaxing effect on the physical level. On the soles of our feet there are many reflex points, each communicating holographically with certain regions in the rest of the body. By walking barefoot, these areas get stimulated. This makes use of foot zone reflex massage, but you can also experience this with a simple massage of the feet.

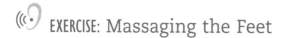 **EXERCISE:** Massaging the Feet

Follow these step-by-step instructions:
- Massage both of your feet, or have someone massage your feet.
- Knead the feet with gentle pressure and strokes, thereby achieving a sense of relaxation.
- You can take a warm foot bath before massaging. It's refreshing, invigorating, and relaxing for the whole body.

Comments and hints: The feet are our interface with the earth and the physical world. With both feet we stand on the earth. Massaging the feet brings attention to the parts of our body that carry us through life. Enjoy the relaxation and strengthen the body's power.

MAKE DECISIONS THAT WORK

To fly as fast as thought, to anywhere that is, you must begin by knowing in advance that you have already arrived.

RICHARD BACH,
JONATHAN LIVINGSTON SEAGULL

Resolving trauma means new levels of brain potential can arise, and new solutions reveal themselves. New circuits can only proceed from relaxation. As long as we are still held in the tension dictated by the long-held dysfunctional pattern, nothing new can develop. There must be time to rest and take a step back. Similarly, you cannot use danger or coercion to force yourself to function. The sense of "I have to work!" will not help.

New ways and new directions presuppose that a decision to heal has been made. Saying what I *don't* want doesn't bring us where we want to go; instead, saying what I *do* want, turning away from what I don't want, makes it possible to achieve that goal.

New circumstances present us with new challenges and sometimes bring new insights—a previously unknown way to solve a problem often emerges. This is exemplified by the following exercise.

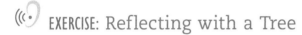 EXERCISE: Reflecting with a Tree

Follow these step-by-step instructions:

- Formulate a question for which you are looking for a solution. It can be the next step in a certain task, or a question about which decision is the right one for you in a particular situation.
- Write the question down on a sheet of paper.
- Read this question aloud once.
- Everything that happens from now on, everything you encounter, may already be an aspect of the answer to your question.
- Go to the woods or to a park and pick out a tree. Welcome the tree like an old friend and sit down with your back to it, with your back facing south (you may need to take a compass with you, or you can use your phone).
- Consider your question first from the feeling side:
  ▸ What emotions does it trigger?
  ▸ How do you respond to your feelings?
- Next, move clockwise 90 degrees. If you started in the south, you will now look toward the west.
  ▸ What or who do you need? This might include certain people with whom you work or who are important for the solution.

- Move clockwise 90 degrees. You will now be facing north.
  - ▸ What is important to learn to study?
  - ▸ What do you not understand?
  - ▸ What knowledge, what information, do you need?
- Move clockwise 90 degrees. You will now be facing east.
  - ▸ Where are you going? What is the most beautiful image you can conjure up for the solution?
  - ▸ How should it be? Imagine the best solution for all parties involved.
- Relax in each direction at least several minutes until you feel that the essential answers to your questions from these four directions have become clear to you, and that it is enough at this time.
- If this is too vague, set a time for each direction; for example, 15 minutes.
- After the last position, you can now say good-bye to your friend the tree.
- Give the tree a small personal gift, for example, a pinch of tobacco (the traditional gift of Native Americans in such rituals in nature) or a few of your hairs.
- Go back to the place where you started.
- Finish the exercise with a big thank you.

Comments and hints: For this exercise it's good to bring along a pen and a notebook to write down your thoughts.

Observe what you encounter from the beginning to the end of the exercise: animals that make their presence known during this meditation, even the smallest ones; characters that crop up in your mind; a special person; or perhaps a slogan that especially stands out to you. Note if any directions around the tree are particularly comfortable or uncomfortable.

The clearer we are about where we want to go, the clearer our thoughts and subsequent actions will be to bring us there. To educate ourselves and to act continuously to achieve the desired goal requires a workout. This is the subject of the next chapter.

9

No Pain, No Gain

Exercises for Resonance,
Regulation, and Repetition

TRAINING BRINGS
KNOWLEDGE TO ACTION

Our body has two halves, a right side and a left side that under optimal conditions operate in balanced interaction. Bringing the two into harmony is a lifelong task. The fact of having two sides in our physical being also has a deeper meaning: different, complementary forces work within us, striving for inner and outer balance.

Different cultures also consider this dualism. In China this principle is expressed by the yin-yang symbol. In the pre-Columbian civilizations of Central America, two intertwined snakes symbolized it. We also find this principle in the caduceus, the staff carried by Hermes in Greek mythology, around which is intertwined two snakes.

These forces are not warring opponents but rather complementary aspects of a single force. This single force is the universal energy responsible for building the basic structures of organisms, such as our perception, that are based on bilateral symmetry. This idea comes from ancient knowledge that says that balance is of fundamental importance in all processes of regeneration. We can regenerate our hearing and bring

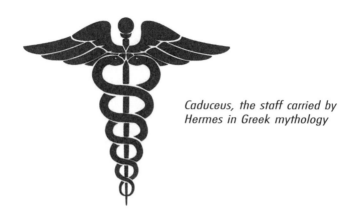

Caduceus, the staff carried by Hermes in Greek mythology

ourselves into balance with training. The task is not to help us handle a hearing deficit better but to restore the underlying order. This is achieved by resolving the experiences that have led to imbalance. Without guidance, the brain is constantly trying to calculate and seeks a starting point from which to **calibrate.** So our first step in restoring the natural order is to correctly locate the sound source in the listening field.

> **Calibrate:** To determine, rectify, or mark the gradations of something; to adjust precisely for a particular function (after the French *calibrer*)

In all learning processes we need to integrate new knowledge into our own world and apply it. When we learn, we build on our experience and our own findings. Only from there can we record new things. Therefore we must proceed in training and developing our listening field in clear, comprehensible steps. It's like that time in school when we learned mathematics. We didn't start immediately with multiplication and square roots but rather with the numbers 1 to 10, then we moved on to larger numbers and more and more complex calculations.

We know from brain research of the existence of mirror neurons.[1] These are neurons that fire both when an animal (such as a human) acts *and* when it observes the same action performed by another. So, when we see or experience something outside of ourselves what we see or experience reflects back inside of us. These special nerve cells can be stimulated for a lifetime and are capable of making new experiences that can be called up at any time.

In each process of perception—acoustic, visual, and **kinesthetic**—mirror neurons are involved in imitating an action. This becomes clearest when the body imitates the action it sees. Imitation is how humans have learned many things.

However, knowledge must be applied in order to integrate the imitation. Through applying the imitation we learn what actually works, and we make our own experiences. This physical feedback motivates us to learn and experience further and leads to eventual success. If I have not used a muscle for a long time, it becomes weak. It hasn't disappeared, it's just weak. But the body can regain strength bit by bit through physical therapy. The same is true for hearing loss. The entire listening system is very much like a muscle that hasn't been used, and bit by bit it can be restored through training.

Kinesthetic: Based on kinesthesia, a sense mediated by receptors located in muscles, tendons, and joints and stimulated by bodily movements and muscle contractions; movement sensitive (Greek, *kinein,* "move," and *aisthesis,* "perception")

EVERYTHING FLOWS

The ancient Greek philosopher Heraclitus asserted that "everything flows" (*panta rhei*). Change is the fundamental essence of the universe; all beings are in a process of becoming. We ourselves and everything around us—everything we see, touch, and feel—has emerged from a process of self-regulation, a process of continuous change and evolution. Life shows us that higher, more complex structures arise from simpler ones. This is only possible because of the self-organizing principle of life, which, although carried out in matter, is not part of matter. It is certainly a *quality* of matter, however. This is immediately perceived in the moment when the spirit or the soul leaves a living being, be it a small beetle, a faithful dog who accompanied us, or a loved one. Without consciousness, the body quickly breaks down.

This shows that all beings have consciousness. Without this, no matter can realize, organize, and come together. This self-organization principle is subject to the effects of any number of forces. Pain, injury, and trauma support decomposition, division, or a split in the organism. Just as a knife splits a loaf of bread, an unkind word divides us. Trauma splits a unity into a multiplicity, leading to **entropy** (in the physical sense), a process of degradation leading to disorder. The Austrian physicist Ludwig Boltzmann (1844–1906) formulated the principle that nature tends from a less probable to a more probable state. The most likely state is always the greatest possible disorder. However, life obviously contradicts this and simple forms such as protozoa eventually develop more complex forms.

> **Entropy:** A measure of the unavailable energy in a closed thermodynamic system that is also usually considered to be a measure of the system's disorder, which is a property of the system's state (thermodynamics); the measure of disorder in a closed system (Greek, *entrepein,* "repent, turn").

The emerging force, the evolutionary force, consists of love and awareness. Awareness means perception and understanding of the parts. If I perceive the individual parts, I understand their relationships and their interaction, which adds to form a whole. For example, if I look at a pile of Lego blocks and see various possibilities in it, I can assemble the blocks into something more complex.

Our lives are full of polarities: light/dark, hot/cold, near/far, good/evil, and many more. We can regard polarities as opposites, but in reality they are aspects of a commonality that contains these parts and out of which the two poles are fed. For example, light/dark is nourished by the light of the sun; hot/cold is nourished by heat energy.

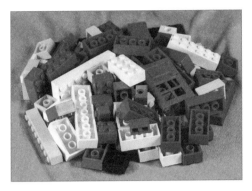

Individual parts show potential.

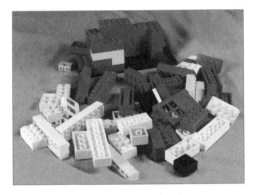

An idea begins to take shape.

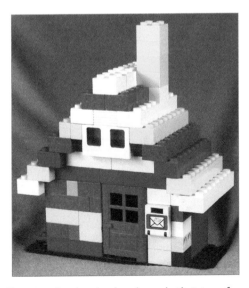

The visualized order has been built into a form.

There is always a single space that encloses everything that is included in it, including the poles. So, if I stimulate both poles simultaneously from the outside—even our body has these two poles—I create an assembly.

In the basic method of hearing regeneration we work with the poles: I can/I can't; stress/relaxation; near/far; loud/quiet. By stimulating both poles, they connect and work together more smoothly, which refines our overall capabilities. So we work with both aspects of a system.

Always remember, if we come to a point where we feel that the process is stalling, that means we are in contact with a traumatic event. The pain of the trauma triggers in us involuntary paralysis, rigidity, and helplessness. To get through the resistance we need movement. The movements in the exercises of the basic method give us physical and mental information that will help us move into and past the trauma toward resolution, but the choice to engage in them is ours.

A walk, a massage, a brief period of rest and relaxation can also help.

THE GOAL IS INTEGRATION

You have to know a lot to do little.
WILLIBALD PSCHYREMBEL,
GYNECOLOGIST AND EDITOR OF THE
GERMAN *CLINICAL DICTIONARY*,
IN REFERENCE TO OBSTETRICS

As we know, the human body is based on certain physical principles and a common basic structure. Your self-regulatory process can lead your body back to its original order, provided that it receives "skillful non**intervention**."

Intervention: The act of interfering with the outcome or course of a condition or process (late Latin, *interventio*, "mediation")

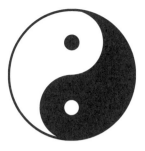

The opposite yet complementary forces of the universe are depicted in the yin-yang symbol of Chinese philosophy.

Consider the yin-yang symbol: much is hidden in this sign. We first see an apparent polarity (light/dark, male/female). In fact, it's not a polarity—the two aspects form a perfect circle, a common space that encloses everything. This is the order of the yin-yang symbol. The next thing we can see is two dots. They represent the static element of our perception. They show that in each part there is an element of the other. The third thing we see is the dynamics of the yin-yang, which is seen as a wavy line, a sinusoid, which represent a full passage or a full cycle.

This symbol is a two-dimensional representation of the interaction between seemingly contradictory forces. A striking resemblance to this ancient symbol is found when looking at a depiction of our cochlea from

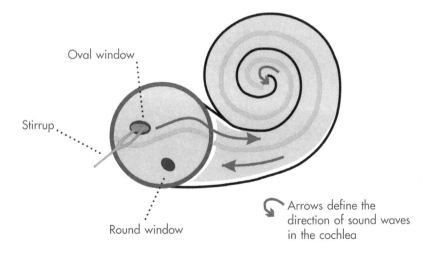

Oval window

Stirrup

Round window

Arrows define the direction of sound waves in the cochlea

The cochlear or cochlea viewed from the outside with a round and oval window

the front. It carries on its surface 2 points in the form of membranes that receive sound pulses in fluid-filled channels. These run in spirals up to a tip, where they are connected and run through a 180-degree rotation back to the beginning.

We always have both static and dynamic elements within us. In the basic therapeutic method, both aspects are present and included. That's one of the reasons why it's so efficient. We have the static element in the form of the static singer or the water noise, which always form a fixed reference point, as does the voice of the partner. And we have the dynamic element of moving through the listening field. That's how we get our system moving so well. When the process is completed, we have experienced two fundamental aspects of our perception: first, the "front," the alignment with the sound source, and then—by turning our back to the therapeutic seat—the "back."

There is yet another interpretation of the yin-yang symbol, something universal and something individual. The symbol indicates a law: All energy moves basically as a sine wave. We do not know of another type of energy movement in our physical universe. Perhaps no other is possible. How energy moves overall is the same for everyone. But how this curve looks in detail—if it has a nicely curved, smooth motion, whether it has sharp spikes, or whether a part is overemphasized—that is individual, because there is no law governing individuals.

This leads us to another exercise.

EXERCISE: Resonance in Movement

Follow these step-by-step instructions:

- In pairs or in a group, the instruction to stand up and then to sit down again is given.
- Do this 5, 10, or 20 times. A resonance will automatically be created and the movements will eventually converge until all participants are more or less in sync.

Comments and hints: If we feel comfortable with the people we're doing this exercise with, a common rhythm is easily found. If not, it's good to talk about how each person felt during this exercise and what they were thinking.

Resonance with one another in an exercise such as this supports the process of regulation.

Rhythm and movement are the beginning of organization within an organism. When an order impulse is brought into the body's systems, then all parts begin to swing back together and communicate in a state of resonance. For example, the kidneys begin to harmoniously resonate with the other organs.

This is not about saying, for example, that the blood pressure is too high or too low but about understanding *why* this specific function has decoupled itself and is in a state of dissonance with the overall system. If I jog, then my blood pressure might rise initially, as my heart is pumping harder—my body knows what is needed to expend this kind of energy. When I'm relaxed, my blood pressure drops again. However, it is not conducive to my overall system if I run and my heart does not cooperate by raising my blood pressure. All components of the system must work together and support one another. The better they work together and support one another, the easier it is for me to implement my goal.

If my legs get tired because I haven't used them in a long time, I have to give my legs time to get back into good form through regular training. It's important to make sure that all the subsystems involved in the movement can work together and feel good, otherwise it places excessive demands on the entire system.

BREAKING DOWN BARRIERS

We all build protective walls and barricades when we experience overwhelming pain or trauma. This is quite natural. To unpack these experiences for reevaluation, the system must be unlocked. By unlocking I refer to the active process of the person undergoing training to let go of existing (and often painful) tension in the body. These tensions have been built around painful events and are comparable to the tension that we experience in the body when we get scared. The basic method supports this release, so that the events of our conscious perception are accessible again in the form of feelings, images, and thoughts.

Because this kind of self-protection around traumatic situations has been established for a reason, there are two tasks involved in unlocking the protection: 1) the initial release to set the processing in motion, and 2) allowing the listener to determine the speed and processing of traumatic experiences according to their own needs; this can be done quickly or slowly depending on the person. The basic therapeutic method ensures self-determination of the process by the listener and does not encourage speeding up by someone other than the listener. Thus it depends on where they are at physically or emotionally. There should be no excessive demands placed on the listener's system; the person experiences the process of change and the steps toward improving their listening field on their own terms, which motivates the person to continue to train. Sometimes the listener may not be ready to allow regulation. This may mean that the person needs more time to dissolve the gradually built-up defensive wall, because regulation means that the person must access the painful events that are the cause of hearing loss. Subconsciously, we feel the pain behind the protective wall and want to avoid it. At this point, however, it is not about forcing anything, but instead allowing the process to unfold naturally.

A central task of our perceptual system is to **duplicate** the external reality inside, to process it. It can feel stressful when the map of external reality no longer matches the map of internal reality.

Duplicate: Being the same as another; a double (Latin, *duplicare*)

Our aim in this work is to resolve the difference between the perception of the outside reality and the perception of the inside reality. Relaxation is the key to ensuring that anything can be resolved. The man who feels that he no longer hears anything becomes tense. Therefore, relaxation is necessary for a new order to take the place of the old pattern. The reorganization of the listener's perception is also felt on the physical level, in that energy throughout the system can flow more smoothly.

The partner in this process is very important. He provides a framework for the listener, through his knowledge and confidence, to allow the listener to proceed. He is there to accompany and support the trainee in this process and provide a sense of security. For us as partners in this process it is important that we lead the listener through the steps and not stop prematurely because we think results aren't coming. We must always follow the trainee in the process, and that includes whether or not the person wants to stop.

REPETITION OF THE EXERCISES

Knowledge cannot be transferred, it can only be created anew in each person's brain. Our souls and our bodies need time to process new impressions and insights. Continuous step-by-step training will help you gradually realize what has hurt you and caused a weakening in your sense of hearing. It is like a field full of stones—we can only remove them one by one. By taking the stones from the field and building a windbreak or a house with them, we remove the obstacles that make it difficult for us to produce food and plants. The same is true for training; our soil lies within us, and the stones are our life experiences. Through them we learn and grow, so they can even empower us in some ways. Through this process of removing the stones of our life we rebuild our listening field.

The exercises in part 2 of this book (considered phase 2 of training), done at home over a period of 8 to 12 weeks, facilitate the integration of new knowledge so that stability and security can develop and become anchored.

It's understood that we will experience some days in which we seem to have trouble hearing even though we've been making overall progress through training. That's where the repetitiveness of the process is helpful in reinforcing our progress, because those days will pass.

That's why after an interval of 2 to 4 weeks the exercises should be repeated again for a few weeks. This sequence—specific training and a pause—should be repeated several times, as it supports our abilities in many ways, for not only our hearing, but our body's balance and power are also strengthened. There is a bit of a temptation that you will quickly see a result and then stop. However, for long-term integration and development of what is learned, it is important to repeat these exercises.

Although some of the exercises in phase 2 require a partner, this is one central exercise that you can do alone, without a partner.

(( )) EXERCISE: Training Solo

First I will explain the exercise with a natural, fixed sound source; thereafter, with the hologram of the Naturschallwandler, a natural sound transducer. This exercise is based on the basic method as described in chapter 5, and it complements the earlier training. For the first part of this exercise you will be working with a running water faucet as a natural, fixed sound source.

Training with a Natural Sound Source
Follow these step-by-step instructions:
- Set up a chair in front of the faucet with the back of the chair facing the tap. This is the therapeutic seat.
- Place a second chair exactly opposite at a distance of approximately 2.5 yards, facing the water source and the therapeutic seat; the distance will subsequently vary from session to session, from 1.5 to 4 yards (as room size allows). The chairs should be stable and should not be moveable (as office chairs are) so as to convey a sense of stability and security. Armrests are good but not necessary.
- Now go to the tap and turn it on slowly until you hear the sound of

water significantly. If the sound is too quiet, increase the volume by placing a pot right-side up or upside down under the faucet, or something else "tinny" that amplifies the sound.

■ Walk to the chair that faces the water source and sit down. Close your eyes while placing both feet side-by-side on the floor. As before, go barefoot or wear socks or slippers.

■ Imagine that the sound of water is in front of you, even if you hear it elsewhere through this part of the exercise, the brain trains the first direction).

■ Now take note of where you actually hear the sound and listen to the sound for 3 to 4 minutes.

■ After a few minutes of listening, stretch out your hand to where you hear the noise.

■ Now open your eyes to check whether your hearing perception is correct (the right place of the sound being directly opposite and to the front).

■ Close your eyes again for about 1 minute.

■ Only if you heard the sound clearly, right in front of you, you can now open your eyes, stand up, and walk slowly toward the therapeutic seat. Turn right in front of the seat and sit down on the chair so that the faucet is at your back. At the same time, remain alert to the sound of the water.

■ If you did not hear the sound of the water clearly, before completing this part of the exercise, start all over again the next day or the day after that.

● If you do continue because you have heard the sound clearly, once you have settled in the therapeutic seat your auditory perception will be correct if you now clearly hear the noise behind you. This is the aim of this exercise.

■ Listen to the sound for about 30 seconds. Then shut off the tap and again sit down in the therapeutic seat for about 2 minutes in silence.

■ Do this exercise regularly about every 2 days.

Comments and hints: If while doing this exercise you think of stressful experiences from your past that are related to hearing, write them down as soon as possible. This helps to create some distance between you and the event. You should use a separate sheet of paper for each experience, adding new recollections over time as they arise. These stressful situations are now more complete and get their proper place in the past.

Training with the Naturschallwandler
Natural Sound Transducer

Follow these step-by-step instructions:

- Set up the therapeutic listening field. Place one therapeutic seat with its back to the equipment. Use the same setup and music as previously described. Place a second chair opposite this seat, facing it, at a distance of approximately 2.5 yards; this distance will vary from exercise to exercise, from 1.5 to 4 yards, as room size allows. The chairs should be stable and shouldn't have wheels, so as to convey a sense of stability and security. Armrests are good but not necessary.

- Now sit down in the seat facing the equipment, pick up the remote control, and close your eyes. Place both feet side-by-side on the floor. It's best to be barefoot, or wear socks or slippers.

- Start the music by remote control. You will begin quietly then slowly increase the volume until you hear the singer well. When you do, set the remote to the side.

- Just imagine now that the singer is in front of you, even if you hear her elsewhere (through this part of the exercise, the brain trains in the first direction).

- Take note of where you actually do hear the singer and extend your hand in that direction.

- Open your eyes to see whether your hearing perception is correct. The place of the singer should be right in front of you, between the two satellites.

- Close your eyes again and continue to listen. You may have to go back to the first track by means of remote control.

- Only if you clearly hear the singer in front of you, open your eyes, stand up, and walk slowly to the therapeutic seat nearer the equipment, turn right in front of the seat, and sit in the chair. The equipment will be at your back. In doing so, your attention should stay with the music.

- If you cannot hear the singer clearly at this point, turn the music volume down with the remote control until it is no longer heard, and then turn off the music. Try doing the exercise again the next day from the beginning.
- If you have heard the singer clearly, once you have settled on the therapeutic seat your auditory perception will be correct if you now clearly hear the singer from behind you. This is the goal of the exercise.
- Listen to the rest of the music, then turn it off.
- To wind down and relax, as well as strengthen your listening field, you can now listen to one or two tracks from the CD *Sources of Healing*, or some other relaxing piece of music.
- Do this exercise regularly about every 2 days.

Comments and hints: If you think of any stressful experiences from your past that are related to your hearing, write them down as soon as possible. This helps to create some distance between you and the event. You should use a separate sheet for each experience, adding new recollections over time as they arise. These stressful situations are now more complete and get their place in the past.

Progress Takes Time

Let's remember that spatial localization and the balancing of the right and left hemispheres—and thus the entire hearing process—has to be learned by the brain. Don't force anything, as this process can take time. If the sound source or the music changes position, "moves," or "jumps," this is actually a good sign of reorientation in ear-brain coordination. It is important that the noise gradually changes its location to the center.

10
Nothing Is Impossible
One Step at a Time

SERIOUS, CHRONIC PATHOLOGIES OF HEARING such as advanced hearing loss, hyperacusis, or intense tinnitus need a strategy for their permanent resolution. This requires *trust,* a word that implies certain landmarks along the way. One of those is motivation.

Motivation is the key to success. Most people with chronic symptoms of hearing loss have developed a passive attitude toward their condition, understanding it as a loss they can do nothing about. We now know this isn't true. Understanding the relationship between hearing loss and trauma, and knowing that the resolution of trauma can lead to a healing of the condition, helps to supply the motivation needed to persevere in the process. Ask yourself the following questions:

- How do your physical symptoms manifest in your life?
- What trauma do you associate with your hearing loss?
- How can it be resolved?
- What do you do in concrete terms? What are the basic methods that support your gaining insight?

New decisions can lead to new experiences. If I continue to do the things the way I've always done them, then there is no room for change. The decision to embark on a new path is a prerequisite for creating new experiences, new knowledge, and new opportunities.

How do we do this? Set reasonable goals. The road to success consists of individual steps. Also, formulate your overall aim. Every step is important. Life itself is a process and not a state, so it's always taking a direction. The immediate goal at first is not to get rid of the symptoms or pain of hearing loss but instead to understand the triggering issue and methodically resolve it step-by-step. As you do this, bring back your inherent listening skills through training and build new possibilities. In this case, the goal is to restore the harmony in the brain back to the way it was before the traumatic event that led to the hearing deficit.

When we have symptoms of hearing loss over a long period, the brain has adapted to this dysfunctional condition and reinforces it based on the principle "use it or lose it." This refers to the neurons that are heavily used to react faster and more intensively to acoustic signals. Acoustic stimuli include hugely magnified sound (hyperacusis) or constantly repeating sound (tinnitus). Therefore, an important point on the path to healing—especially at moments when the symptoms are particularly strong—is to do positive activities that have nothing to do with the symptom to strengthen the mental skills to change the pain networks in the brain. Passively waiting until the acute stress is over brings no change. This is not about stress or distraction. It's about teaching your system, when overloaded, to use the neural networks to connect with positive impulses.

An example of such a positive activity is to use visualization. Imagine how it is when the symptoms decrease as the brain shuts down the dysfunctional signal, so to speak—like a dimmer that regulates the intensity of the light. Other positive activities might include treating yourself to a soothing massage, playing a musical instrument, cooking something good, writing a story, juggling, going on a pleasant run, doing tai chi, jumping on a trampoline, playing soccer with children, or just doing something physical, whatever it is that you enjoy. *It is important that your activity brings about pleasant physical sensations.* This is a process that takes time and a fair amount of discipline, especially to go on even if you're not yet seeing any positive results. Through the basic

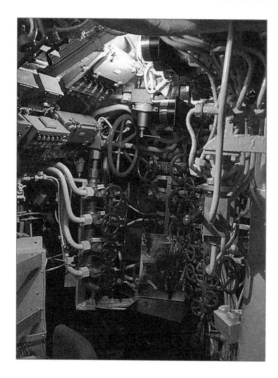

*Change the brain circuitry
to make new connections.*

therapeutic method we rebuild our original skills that have been lost
and process the cause of the hearing disorder. It's about gaining knowledge, not repressing it. When we experience pain, we sometimes try to
push back or endure and perhaps distract ourselves (with activities such
as work). This is not a good approach.

Recent findings on **neuroplasticity** show that significant empha-
sis must be placed on changing the brain circuits and making new
connections. Resist the temptation to divert your attention from the
condition, because such diversions only reinforce and strengthen the
old circuits in the brain. It takes perseverance and consistency to
make new connections. This means confronting pain and recognizing
the facts.

Neuroplasticity: The ability of synapses, nerve cells, or entire
areas of the brain to change, depending on their use (Greek,
neuron, "tendon, nerve," and *plastikos,* "to form"). The brain of an

adult is not a rigid, fixed organ, but rather it changes constantly, even into old age. New experiences and impressions change the architecture of the brain, build connections between nerve cells, and build bridges to existing knowledge, while little or unused connections are weakened.[1]

Repetition brings order and stability. One should not stop until there are results. Reliability generates strength and confidence. The brain is constantly trying, like any living system, to find a balanced, peaceful, actionable state. The problem is that sometimes it reaches a situation where the unconscious and automated systems are not sufficient to resolve a brain-body problem such as chronic pain. In this case we must provide conscious control. The control consists of renewed and conscious learning until the brain and body can continue without this conscious input—until self-regulation takes effect. Repetition anchors the new capability, as the brain circuits are rebuilt or restrengthened.

Repetition: A motion or exercise that is repeated (Latin, *repetitio,* "to repeat")

Our task is to free the brain from repeating the same thoughts and patterns again and again. If we feel that the pain doesn't stop, the side effect is fear because we see no end in sight. The feeling of anxiety is amplified because pain in the body turns on the **amygdala.** This area is centrally located in the brain and is responsible for analyzing the potential risk of external stimuli and choosing (albeit unconsciously) necessary reactions. It also influences the release of stress hormones and the **vegetative** nervous system.[2]

Amygdala: A paired core area of the brain, part of the limbic system that primarily serves the processing the development of instinctive responses (Greek, *amygdale,* "almond")

Vegetative: Unconscious, not lying with the will; dull, monotonous, passive (late Latin, *vegetatus,* past participle of *vegetare,* "to live, grow")

Chronic pain, hyperacusis, and even tinnitus have their causes in the past. However, the pain is in the present. Due to the repetition of the same processes in the brain the dysfunctional pattern is constantly being strengthened. Therefore, chronic pain is also learned pain. The amygdala is the brain structure responsible for the emotional coloration of information. Therefore, it is important to face the pain and recognize the cause. On one hand what burdens us presently and on the other hand what has hurt us in the past could not be resolved at that time, so the task is to dissolve fixed circuits by finding a solution today for what was not solvable at the time when the painful event happened. By understanding what weighs on us, we can find a way to end this burden and thus resolve the pain. That's the job.

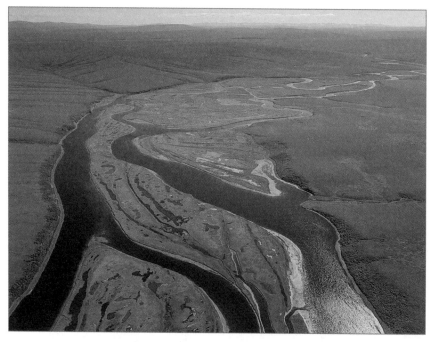

Over time, nature constantly changes, creating new pathways.

We must stay flexible and open in the case of resistance; we must recognize the pain and process it. Not only do we want to feel better, but we also want to restore normal brain function. This isn't about temporary relief but about a longer process of deep regulation. To do that, we need to persevere and recognize that small, steady progress is a sign that the previously rigid system is moving and changing.

Finally, we must build our energy by recognizing what's good for us and abandoning what we don't want. Without energy, we can't implement anything; we will have no strength for change and new developments. You can restore your natural way of being. Each person is unique. Find your essence.

Here's a wonderful exercise that you already know that restores energy.

EXERCISE: Walking, the Basic Movement of Life

Follow these step-by-step instructions:

- The secret is to go slowly. Find your own rhythm and align your body.
- In the beginning go walking 3 times a week for 5 minutes on level ground after 5 minutes of gentle warm up exercises.
- Walk with gentle movements while using your arms, all in a fluid motion. Find your own rhythms. It's not about going as far or as long as possible, but to consciously carry out the movements of the body: the movement of the feet and legs, as you set the foot down and pick it back up; the movement of the arms; the posture of the upper body; the alignment of the head with the spine . . .
- Gradually extend this exercise to more days of the week until it becomes a daily ritual.
- The routes you take can change, sometimes going over rough terrain or going up and down stairs.
- After walking slowly, walk at your usual pace

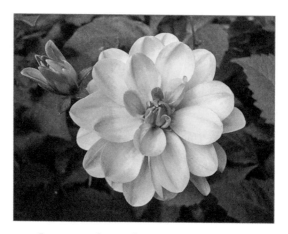

Beauty, a shining beacon in the darkness

Comments and hints: This exercise is therefore the next stage of the exercise called "Walking Straight Ahead," which was described in chapter 6. Training our sense of balance by moving over rough terrain and up and down stairs is part of this exercise. By slowing down the movement, the major muscles of this action are addressed, as well as the muscles for the fine control of movement. You will probably feel muscles you would otherwise hardly have noticed by starting out slowly.

THE APPROACH OF CONVENTIONAL MEDICINE AND THE FAILURE OF HEARING AIDS

To face pain means to learn more about it. Perhaps for a long time we hoped something would happen to alleviate the pain so we'd get better again. Finally, we decided to go to the doctor. We wanted to know about the cause of the pain and find out what we could do about it. It is useful to be clear about the facts: on the one hand, we may have had a traumatic event, an accident, or an illness that led to a more or less severe hearing loss; and on the other hand, we may have experienced more gradual hearing loss that is usually explained by old age or life circumstances, such as work-related stress.

Even if the facts are sobering or frightening, how a doctor communicates those facts can make a big difference. Many doctors today have a tendency to give the worst-case scenario so that the patient doesn't get false hope and is disappointed when conventional therapeutic measures are not successful. There is, of course, nothing wrong with getting a medical diagnosis. However, when you open the door to the possibility of a positive change, you are beginning the process of self-regulation and true healing. Just because you've had no experience with alternative methods doesn't mean there can't be improvements and that the last word has been spoken. Even if the functional mechanisms of my ear have been destroyed—which is actually very rare in reality—I still have a second ear. I know that each ear is cross-connected in both hemispheres. This gives me an opportunity to build a functional listening field through training, so that I can move comfortably and safely through my world.

Even when there's been severe damage in the inner ear, particularly in the cochlea (see page 17), where connections are broken or appear to not function, there is still a rudimentary receiving system in place in the form of the eardrum, ear bones, and cochlea. So before we conclude that no improvement is possible, it's very important to take the time to examine what can still perhaps be achieved with the existing reception system. Therefore, it should be repeatedly pointed out that just because the classic medical opinion says it's impossible, each person is unique and contains a natural self-healing ability. So let's not jump to conclusions too quickly and assume that nothing can be done and that we just have to accept our fate.

Hearing is primarily a process of information processing in the brain. Of course, the mechanical parts of the ear also play an important role, but the central role of everything that is involved in the hearing *process* is often underestimated. Our brain is capable of obtaining a complete picture from just a few pieces of information. If I see an image that consists of only a few pixels, I can still recognize who the person is if I know them. If I see a simple picture painted by a child, I can say, "This is Mom, Dad, and Sis."

We can make a complete scenario out of incomplete information. This is all the more possible if I have a clear reference point from which I can build the whole picture. For example, if the hairs in my ear are damaged, they are not dead but rather receive less information. Maybe even some of the hairs are no longer functioning, but all of them? We have about 30,000 of them in our inner ear. Do we really know that we have irreparable damage to the hearing organ? "This is just the way it is" is often said, but in fact we do not know for sure. It makes a big difference whether I think, *This is just the way it is,* versus *We might have some damage to the cochlea.* Of course, there is damage or a weakening as evidenced by the fact that we don't hear so well anymore, but does that mean there's nothing more to be done, that the situation cannot improve? Some of the hairs may be damaged, some may only be bent, and some might be just fine. This is similar to having a weak signal— the signal still carries the complete information, it's just weak. When I learn how to deal with this weak signal, then I can have fuller hearing and more complete perception. I can understand again what is happening acoustically around me.

That's why conventional medicine's diagnostic model of broken hairs with related hearing loss is not wrong, but instead we should ask, "How can I learn to hear better again?" The approach of conventional medicine is basically to reinforce the external noise with a hearing aid, making it a lot louder. But with this solution we don't improve our internal processing, we simply increase the pressure on the organ. This "make it louder" approach that requires a hearing aid means that the spatial localization process and the internal order will not be rebuilt. The hearing aid sends a direct sound pulse into the ear, making everything louder, regardless of where the sound is coming from. Through this purely technical manipulation, no matter where the sound is coming from it is sent to my ear, and always from the same direction. So

I cannot learn how to retrain my listening capability. Of course, trying to improve the mechanism of hearing, the organ itself, is good, but the hearing aid cannot replace the complex process that constitutes our natural acoustic sense, and in the end it will not bring the improvement we had hoped for. This is certainly one of the reasons why 60 percent of all hearing aids end up in a drawer.[3]

The increasing weakness of our hearing brings up strong feelings of loss. People who already wear one or even two hearing aids usually have an odyssey behind them. Nobody wants to wear a hearing aid. But at some point you can't hear well enough anymore, and so the doctor recommends a hearing aid as a last resort. Inwardly, people are usually resistant to the idea and decline the recommendation, but then they come to the realization that they just can't hear well enough and resign themselves to using a hearing aid.

A hearing aid is like a crutch. If there is no other way, then it's helpful, no question about it. It's not an either-or. But doesn't it make sense to find out if I really need the crutch, and *when* I need it? Is it possible to learn how to hear again through training and to experience a subsequent strengthening? Of course, that is exactly the premise of our approach to restoring hearing naturally.

Natural Regeneration through Changes in Life

Hearing can be regenerated without special training, sometimes simply by the fact that the living conditions have changed, as reported by a professional musician, Martin Ortner. He wrote to me on August 7, 2017:

Dear Mr. Stucki,

My acoustic stress began when I was just 15 years old, when I was relatively close to entering my professional orchestra studies, after participating in various musical ensembles that placed a heavy burden on my hearing, as you can well imagine.

At the age of 21, in 1976, I earned my first fixed commitment with the Vienna Volksoper. The seating arrangement in the orchestra pit was at that time fixed, as opposed to today when every conductor can determine his own seating arrangement for the orchestra. Thus, the viola group sat on the right of the conductor, directly in front of the trumpets (behind which was the percussion section). The noise of the orchestra was usually loudest in the finale of an opera or operetta. Even for a young musician, it was a great physical and psychological stress, as you can imagine. It was particularly stressful for me because behind us sat the percussion section with cymbals and timpani, as well as the almost unbearable piccolo and the entire brass section, which can make an orchestra sound incredibly loud.

In recent years I have only been able to play with specially made silicone earplugs.

By the time I retired on April 1, 2016, I had received a hearing aid, which was generously funded by the Health Insurance Institute. It was preceded, of course, by a specialist medical hearing test, which was confirmed by the Hearing Institute. I must confess that I rarely used the hearing aid right from the beginning. It was so annoying for me.

After almost exactly a year, I had my hearing tested again, and after comparing the results of the two tests it turned out that my hearing had apparently regenerated, and in various high frequencies, so that the hearing aid is now completely unnecessary for me.

I hope to have served you with my letter.

Yours sincerely,

Professor Martin Ortner

Regardless of how sophisticated it may be, the hearing aid is always a strain on our hearing, as our ears get an immediate and direct sound impulse. Filtering and ordering, as occurs in natural hearing, isn't possible for any kind of reasonable price in a hearing device. A hearing aid cannot know from which direction the squeal of tires is coming from and whether it's close by or far away.

If a sound isn't correctly assigned a location, it becomes a burden on our brain. Without the ability to spatially locate, people become disoriented and tense up because they cannot clearly "see" where a sound is coming from. They are often frightened when somebody suddenly comes to them from an unexpected side. Because a hearing aid cannot perform this spatial localization function—and this has nothing to do with the quality of the device—people abandon it almost as soon as they get one. Of course, if I hear almost nothing, a hearing device will provide some improvement because at least now I can perceive sounds that I previously couldn't hear at all—but it's still a great burden on my brain. That's why reducing this burden, through training, makes sense.

This view is contrary to the view of many conventional medical doctors, particularly hearing professionals. They will tell you that you should just get used to the hearing aid, and get one as soon as possible, because your hearing could get much worse otherwise. Deciding what you want to do is a personal choice, of course, and you should take your time in making it. Meanwhile, it's good to know there may be other options.

TRAINING FOR HEARING AID USERS

By training with a natural sound source like running water or a natural sound transducer such as the Naturschallwandler, it is possible to raise the hearing threshold again, so that a hearing aid is no longer needed. The aim is to entirely dispense with the hearing aid. This can be a lengthy process that requires continuous commitment. During training, having to frequently switch back and forth from using a hearing aid to not using one, as sometimes occurs with those who have significant hearing loss, is often difficult because your system cannot adjust to the natural and unreinforced state of hearing, which is an added challenge. Depending on the degree of hearing loss, the use of a hearing aid outside training might be necessary. Meanwhile, if the basic hearing test is given without a hearing aid—that is, I can hear in a one-on-one conversation—it makes sense then to have the device with you during training just in case you feel the need to wear it.

The following is a conversation I had with Mrs. B., born in 1939, which I recorded. Before I started recording, we talked about her fears and what is possible and what isn't, and how hearing affects our reality and determines our lives. At this point Mrs. B. had been training intensively for some time with the Naturschallwandler on her own (see pages 232 to 233).

A Successful At-Home
Story of Regeneration

Mrs. B.: *Since training, I suddenly notice little things again. It started with boiling water. This effervescence, I can now hear again. I also hear knocking again, which before was just a flat-like sound. Right now I have my hearing aids in while talking to you, but I usually don't wear them because I can hear sounds I couldn't hear before.*

Anton: *To me, it is crucial that you have started training by yourself.*

Mrs. B.: *What else can possibly change? But I also got guidance from Mrs. H. [a hearing tech trained by Anton Stucki] that was important.*

Anton: *What was that?*

Mrs. B.: *Mrs. H. knows the developmental steps for the procedure when you do it alone; she knows them exactly. As a lay person you don't know them. That was very helpful. Right now I can work on training on my own. I don't need a guide because the procedure runs in me!*

Anton: *It's important to get out of the downward spiral of thinking there will be no change, and then you realize, "Ah, something changed," and a new way of thinking and feeling begins.*

Mrs. B.: *The world has expanded for me again. Last year, I couldn't participate in a course I enrolled in; I canceled it at noon on the first day. I was sitting right next to the speaker but I couldn't hear anything. Then I thought,* No, I'm not doing this any longer, I'll go back to the hotel—that's it. *It was a very emotional experience, but I made this drastic decision. I went back home, though it was actually a letdown. But it was also, for me, a kind of wake-up call: if I couldn't go on without hearing, I couldn't participate in society. Then you came here in the fall. Coincidence? No, a stroke of luck!*

With my tablet, I found you and even though I did not understand everything you said back then I decided I had to try!

THE IMPORTANCE OF SETTING GOALS

A hearing aid amplifies sounds that are close by more than sounds that are further away. That is why a hearing aid is more supportive in situations where it is loud outside. It is important that we feel secure and safe.

Wearing a hearing aid is similar to when you have a broken leg and then must walk on crutches. At some point you have to stop using the crutches and learn normal walking again. You may feel a bit shaky in the beginning. It's the same with hearing without a hearing aid if you've been using one, and it's important to go through that shaky phase while your system is relearning how to listen. So during this transitional time it is recommended that you always have your hearing aid nearby for security, so that if you do need it it's right there with you.

As a practitioner or a partner helping someone through the exercises, again and again, we have to face our own fears and those of the people with whom we work. When they experience an improvement they may fear that their hearing will get worse again. They are afraid that they will hope again only to be disappointed when the hearing loss returns. This may cause them to not want to begin. Guidebooks, be they by laymen or professionals, may say that hearing loss could get much worse if you do not operate immediately or intervene technically.

Our answer is not "do not worry" or any other form of appeasement. Or worse: "Our system is better than what you know." It's not about putting people under even more pressure. In the end, people should believe in the method they choose to help them restore their hearing.

We can withdraw at any step. You may need to open the space and give the opportunity for the person to decide for himself alone what he wants to do. And once a decision has been made, don't say, "Who says A must also say B." Every decision can be reevaluated at any point.

It is only important that a decision is made in self-determination and out of responsibility for the self. Once the energy begins to flow, you can feel quickly and clearly: Is that right, and what do I do now? When you realize your choice no longer feels correct, a new choice is made.

Chronic physical symptoms of a hearing deficit like hyperacusis, especially if it's been going on for a long time and has only gotten worse with the years, have their own long background story. In cases like these there is a series of cascading events: a triggering event, and then another and another. The accumulated weight of all these events is heavier and more oppressive. Because of the amount of stored-up emotional baggage, we can't realistically expect instant results. The best approach is to gradually build up one's knowledge and insights during training and always remember that the possibility of recovery is definitely within us.

At the same time there are different ways to get to your destination. It's not necessarily a question of defining the ultimate goal. Sometimes we limit ourselves when we try to articulate something too specifically about the future based on what we know now, so we put it more generally: "I want to hear better again," or "I want to talk to my grandchildren at our family reunions again, even when they're noisy." The main issue is whether you think your goal is at all possible. That's why it's important to work at it until you feel, *Yes, I can do this—I can reach this goal!* Setting small, incremental goals for yourself and achieving them will allow you to develop confidence in the method and the fact that you can heal. However, if we don't get closer to a target that is too large, it might incur frustration and doubt.

When setting goals it's also important not to be too fixated on a definite timeline, such as "by next summer," or "by the next family reunion." That automatically generates the kind of pressure you don't want to put on yourself. Instead, formulate a more attainable goal as you work through the process, feel comfortable with that, get to work, and leave the rest to your body's innate self-regulating mechanism. It is said that a journey of a thousand miles begins with a single step. Ultimately, you have to ask yourself this: Between where I am now and my ultimate goal, what is the first step (then the next one, and the one after that, etc.)? What will help me feel satisfied that I am making progress along the way? What is something that will strengthen me and yet be a small enough goal that I absolutely know that I can achieve it?

Here are some other suggestions for working with goals:

- *Agree on verifiable and clear objectives:* If you are a partner in the method, make sure that the person with whom you are working remains realistic and considers the achievement of his or her goals possible.

- *Clarify the foundation for working jointly:* The training partner and the trainee should have open communication with the common goal of developing solutions to inner conflicts that are not yet or not completely dissolved.

- *Make clear financial and time agreements:* Both the person with their issues, as well as the training partner are responsible for clarifying all arrangements concerning time and money, if there is to be financial compensation involved. It makes sense to discuss these matters before beginning any work together.

- *Clearly state your goals and celebrate them when achieved at each step along the way:* If an intermediate goal has been reached, don't start a new level of training on the same day; instead give yourself time so that what you've learned can be integrated and celebrated.

IN THE HERE AND NOW, EASILY

The ear is the way to the heart.

MADELEINE DE SCUDÉRY

In the end, working with the basic method is about helping ourselves and others come to the here and now with their conscious perception. We achieve this through concentration and focus. Supported through personal contact, touch, and accompaniment. Insights, changes, and solutions to old problems can only be discovered in the here and now, in the present—not in the past and not in the future. Therefore, it is important that we come to the present, even when we talk about the past. How do I feel about it *now*? What am I thinking *now*? What do I need to resolve *now*? If we had had the solution earlier, we would not have had work to do.

Being in the moment is enormously strengthened by reading out loud. The following exercise, the last in this book, teaches us to listen to one another and especially to ourselves—so let's listen to our inner voice!

 ## READING OUT LOUD

This exercise can be done alone, at home. Follow these step-by-step instructions:

- Take a book—a book of poetry or prose or anything else you like—and read aloud from it to the sound of running water from a tap or to the sound of music playing on the Naturschallwandler natural sound transducer.
- Take a different position in your listening field, directly in front of the noise source as well as farther away, as well as both inside and outside the sound hologram.

- Vary the volume of your own voice as you read: 1 to 2 minutes quietly without straining your voice, then louder, then even louder, interspersing with reading quietly.
- Vary the volume of the sound source every 5 minutes.
- Finish the exercise immediately when it becomes tiring, or after about 15 minutes.
- Do this exercise about every 3 days until you can hear your voice well with slightly louder sound coming from the natural sound source—both farther away and very near.
- The goal is to hear your own voice well without being affected by the external noise.

Comments and hints: Read a story to other people—especially with children, as this is a nice shared experience. This strengthens our hearing via bone conduction. Hearing your own voice as you read out loud is an aspect of perception by which you can regulate the volume and pitch of your voice and train your hearing. As well, reading aloud is a complex process that supports other functions. The brain must automatically coordinate muscles for speaking, perceive the recognition of words on a page, and process those words as you listen to yourself. This requires focus and increases your ability to concentrate and formulate thoughts.

11
A New Beginning
Four Principles
for a Successful Life

WE HAVE COME A LONG WAY TOGETHER. Thank you for trusting me to present this information, and most of all thank you for having the confidence in yourself to undertake this journey with me. You have gone the full route and have reviewed your own experiences, drawn your own conclusions, and perhaps experienced some ups and downs. Always remember that the only constant is change.

We can strive for better at any time in life, which reminds me of the wonderful story *The 100-Year-Old Man Who Climbed Out the Window and Disappeared.*[1] It doesn't really matter how old we are, where we are, or how far we have come, we can still set goals and take the steps toward reaching them.

What are your life goals? Whatever they are, strive to achieve them!

In Glenda Green's inspirational book *Love Without End,*[2] I found the following four principles that summarize the work that I have presented to you and the core message underlying our work. In my own words, these are:

- *Be the love that you are.* What do you like to do in life? That's a good indication of how your particular special being expresses itself. You are the center of your own life. This view affects the way you think and how you act in the world. *Am I the woman, am I the man that I want to be?* Don't compare yourself to others—this is about what you feel inside yourself. *How far have I come? How close am I to what I feel drawn to?* Only you can know and realize the answers to these questions.

■ *Do the right thing.* The philosopher Immanuel Kant put it this way: "Act only according to that maxim whereby you can, at the same time, will that it should become a universal law." In other words, do you stand behind what you think and do? Not from the perspective of the prevailing morality or ethics—this may change in the course of time—but out of your own sense of what is ethical? Imagine that you are the queen or king of your world and don't need to be accountable to anyone. What would you say? What would you do? The right thing may be a great project that allows you to express yourself fully and honestly, or the right thing may just be helping a neighbor cut the hedge. There are always lots of things we can undertake, so we need to realize we can't do everything. Choose the right thing and then follow through with consistency and direction.

■ *Follow life.* Everything that lives will one day die. This makes life precious; a spiritual warrior sees his inevitable death as his constant adviser. The warrior is a man or a woman who seeks self-knowledge and freedom and knows that this is a lifelong struggle. The spiritual warrior is not a soldier, not a recipient of orders. He does not waste time in self-pity but instead uses the time allotted to follow life. He does not depend on superfluous things, his own vanity, or ineffective structures, ideas, and concepts. He tests himself in terms of his growth.

It makes sense to deal with the past and to honor it. But we can't control our lives looking through a rearview mirror. What is given to us now, in the present, is of enormous value. Knowledge and traditions are our roots. They can bind us or they can be the seeds from which we express our life. Our wisdom and experience add to the development of the whole. Children renew the previous generations' accumulation of wisdom with vitality and purpose; they fulfill what we have set in motion. When it comes to decisions, we need only ask: Does this promote living or dying? Often both are mixed together. Let's focus on living. If we follow life and living, we will instinctively do the right thing, and if we do the right thing, then we are the love that we express. The principles flow into each other.

- *Forgive.* By forgiving, we leave behind everything in the past that has done us no good. There is no point in getting stuck in things that are not going well or things that others have done to us. You have to forgive yourself for the mistakes you've made, and you have to forgive others for theirs. At the same time we should take care and assure that others no longer harm us or the people in our own family, the people in the neighborhood, and far beyond. Seen from a great distance, we all live in one house, our common home— Earth. Through constantly feeling anger, we keep the connection to something or someone who did us no good, or abandoned or betrayed us. It burdens and distracts us from what we carry inside ourselves. If souls were cars, then a vindictive soul would look like an old scrap heap rattling down the road and carrying or pulling all kinds of unnecessary cargo. Life can be measured in terms of its ease, freedom, and activity. Children often display these qualities. They follow the flow of life, living instinctively, and do the right thing without thinking about it. Harmony between intelligence and forgiveness is an aspect of forgiveness.

Simply forgetting doesn't make forgiveness complete, but understanding what went wrong and how it came about does. Usually something goes wrong because an understanding, a willingness, or an ability was incomplete. By simply forgetting, nothing is solved and those unresolved issues keep repeating themselves. Also, you can only really let go of your grudge when you have realized the part you played.[3]

Forgiveness is not about sacrificing yourself. Nor is it an act of passive self-abandonment or resistance-free acceptance of abuse. It's about the release of attachment and blockages, which clears the way for constructive justice.

In all this is the opportunity to start over. Tomorrow I must not be who I am today. We can change our life, and we can even change ourselves, and with that our world will not be as it has been so far.

Thank you for listening to me, and I wish you luck and success on your journey.

Appendix A
Directory of Exercises

THE WAY IN WHICH THE EXERCISES ARE ORDERED follow a process that supports our system to rebuild our sense of hearing and develop its original capabilities again. In practice, the exercises convey the feeling of regulation so you can experience what regulation means and how it works. Each exercise will have a different effect on each person; some may be very effective, others not at all. Find out what works best for you. In all of these exercises, it's not about fitness (although some of them physically strengthen the body) or training a very specific skill. It's about improving the proper functionality of the body. By this I mean that our wonderful body lets us experience what we need to learn. Making this possible without pain and the competitive need to achieve is important if we are to release blockages and regain our original skills.

Take notes on your observations and the results of each exercise. This will be a kind of diary that records your developments and changes.

If an exercise is particularly difficult, then resume later, or the next day or the day after that. Force nothing; always follow your own gut feelings. Exercises that you find particularly strengthening may be done regularly, perhaps as part of a personal training program.

Most exercises should be executed with a natural sound source or, if available, with a Naturschallwandler natural sound transducer to support the impulse for order.

Many of the exercises are done in pairs (listener and partner). It is very important to respect each other's boundaries.

Following are the exercises with details on where you can find them in this book.

Playing Hide-and-Seek, page 26

How Well Do I Hear?, page 41

Flying across a Meadow with Arms Outstretched, page 57

Hearing Someone from Behind, page 64

Bending Back and Forth, page 68

Working with a Mirror, page 70

Breathing Consciously, page 102

The Basic Therapeutic Method Using a Natural Sound Source, page 131

The Basic Therapeutic Method Using a Natural Sound Transducer, page 158

Perceiving a Sound with All the Senses, page 194

Walking Straight Ahead, page 196

Balance and Control, page 198

Finding the Triggering Event, page 203

Blindfolded Identification of Sounds and Their Location, page 207

Get Up and Sit Down, page 212

Massaging the Feet, page 216

Reflecting with a Tree, page 217

Resonance in Movement, page 226

Training Solo, page 230

Walking, the Basic Movement of Life, page 239

Reading Out Loud, page 250

Appendix B
Reproducible Templates

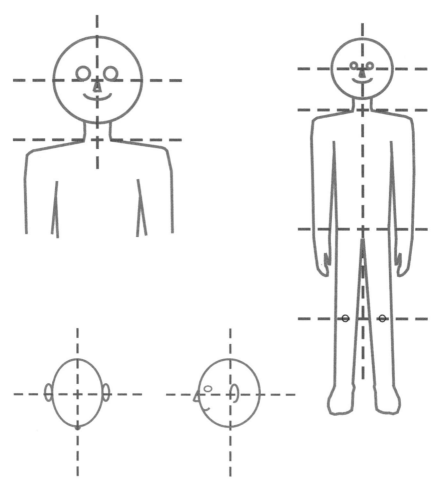

References

BELOW YOU WILL FIND INFORMATION on the sources referenced in this book. All of these sources have inspired me in my life and work—people with their particular expertise and unique approach, innovators who have dared to blaze new trails.

I used to think that a single idea, a single viewpoint, would not be correct for me if I didn't want to explore *all* the works of that author in my field of interest. Today I see things differently. I don't have to agree with everything that an author puts forward; rather, I can take some aspects from that author and apply only those that work for my life and my way of being in the world. There are many other works that I have found valuable over the years that are not specifically cited below but are no less valuable. In this regard I would like to thank all those who have passed on their knowledge in the form of the written word; their findings are a source of inspiration for all of us.

INTRODUCTION

1. Johann Sebastian Bach, *Auf der Suche nach kryptischen Botschaften* [On a search for cryptic messages]. Deutschlandradio [Germany radio], broadcast on March 21, 2014.
2. Michael Stelzner, *Die Symbolik der Zahlen. Die gemeinsamen Gesetze hinter Geist und Materie* [The symbolism of the numbers. The common

law behind spirit and matter] (Wiesbaden: Verlag für außergewöhnliche Perspektiven [Publishing for unusual perspectives], 1997), 25.

3. Friedrich Weinreb, *Schöpfung im Wort—Die Struktur der Bibel in jüdischer Überlieferung* [Creation in the word: the structure of the Bible in Jewish tradition] (Weiler im Allgäu, Germany: Thauros Verlag, 1989), 73.

CHAPTER 1.
A GREAT START MEANS KNOWING
WHERE YOU'RE GOING

1. Rupert Sheldrake, *A New Science of Life* (London: Icon Books, 1981); Rupert Sheldrake, *Das schöpferische Universum. Die Theorie des morphogenetischen Feldes* (Berlin: Ullstein, 1983).
2. "12 Hirnnerven—Basiswissen für jeden Mediziner" [Cranial nerves—Basic knowledge for every physician], *Lecturio Magazine* website, Feburary 19, 2018; "Hirnnerven" neuro24 website [Karl C. Mayer's website about cranial nerves]; "Nerv (Nervus) vestibulocochlearis," medizin kompakt website; John T. Povlishock, "Auditory System," Virginia Commonwealth University e-curriculum website; "Hörbahn," DocCheck Medical Services GmbH website.
3. See "Arbeitsschutz Tabelle Schallpegel Einheiten" [Workplace safety tables of sound-level units], HUG Technik website.
4. "Tontechnik Rechner" [Volume calculator], sengpiel audio website.
5. Peter Tomkins and Christopher Bird, *The Secret Life of Plants* (New York: Harper, 1989 [1973]). German: *Das geheime Leben der Pflanzen* (Frankfurt a. M.: Fischer, 2017).
6. Peter Plichta, *God's Secret Formula* (Rockport, Mass.: Element, 1997). German: *Gottes geheime Formel.* (Munich, Germany: Langen Müller, 1995), 253.

CHAPTER 2.
RETURN TO THE CENTER

1. Petra Jansen-Osmann, "Der Mozart-Effekt–Eine wissenschaftliche Legende?" [Study on the Mozart effect] *Musik-, Tanz- und Kunsttherapie* 17, no. 1 (2006): 1–10.

CHAPTER 3.
OUR DESIRE TO HEAR AND FEEL

1. Joachim-Ernst Berendt, lecture in Psychofonie Symposium, University of Zurich, November 27, 1999.
2. See "Cochlea," DocCheck Medical Services GmbH website.
3. Alfred Tomatis, *The Conscious Ear,* trans. Stephen Lushington, ed. Billie M. Thompson (Barrytown, N.Y.: Station Hill Press, 1991), 186; German: *Das Ohr und das Leben* (Olten, Switzerland: Walter (Patmos), 1995), 317.
4. "Tinnitus sonstige hoerbeeintraechtigungen" [Tinnitus and other health claims], Tinnitus-Liga website, accessed November 16, 2017.
5. "Wir über uns" [About us], Deutscher Schwerhörigenbund (DSB) website.
6. "HNO–hals–nasen–oren, Loch im Trommelfell" [throat–nose–ears, hole in the eardrum], Chirurgie portal website.
7. See "Ohrgeräusche: Tinnitus richtig behandeln" [Ringing in the ears: handling tinnitus properly], Apotheken Umschau website.

CHAPTER 4.
EVERYTHING HAS A BEGINNING

1. Hans Cousto, *The Cosmic Octave* (Mendocino, Calif.: LifeRhythm, 2000 [1987]). German: *Die kosmiche Oktave* (Essen, Germany: Synthesis, 1984), 207 and following.
2. Wendy Doniger O'Flaherty, *The Rig Veda: An Anthology* (New York: Penguin, 1981), mandala 10, hymn 129, verse 2. For this book's German edition, the author quoted Peter Michel, ed., *Rig-Veda—Das heilige Wissen Indiens* [Rig Veda—the sacred knowledge of India] vol. 2 (Wiesbaden, Germany: Marix, 2008), 360, second verse.
3. Masaru Emoto, *Messages from Water* (Japan: Hado, 1999). German: *Die Botschaft des Wassers* (Burgrain, Germany: Koha, 2010).
4. "Das Wichtigste über die Alzheimer-Krankheit" [The most important thing about Alzheimer's disease], Deutsche Alzheimer Gesellschaft website.
5. Tomatis, *The Conscious Ear* [in German: *Das Ohr und das Leben*].

CHAPTER 6.
BEING IN THE PRESENT
TO PROCESS THE PAST

1. Deutschlandradio [Germany radio], December 10, 2014.
2. Theodor Schwenk, *Sensitive Chaos: The Creation of Flowing Forms in Water and Air,* 2nd ed., trans. Olive Whicher and Johanna Wrigley, revised by J. Collis 1996 (East Sussex: Sophia Books, 1965), 28–29.

CHAPTER 8.
EACH SHIP HAS A HELMSMAN

1. The explanations about the brain stem come primarily from notes on July 29, 2015, from the lecture of Gerald Huether in Bad Belzig, Germany.

CHAPTER 9.
NO PAIN, NO GAIN

1. "Spiegelneuronen" [Mirror neurons], Planet Wissen broadcast July 11, 2014.

CHAPTER 10.
NOTHING IS IMPOSSIBLE

1. "Neuroplastizität" [Neuroplasticity], *Online Lexikon für Psychologie und Pädagogik* [Online encyclopedia of psychology and education].
2. "Amygdala," Spektrum website.
3. Pirmin Bossart, "Jetzt hören Sie mal gut zu" [Now you listen to me well], *Luzerner Zeitung* online, April 30, 2017.

CHAPTER 11.
A NEW BEGINNING

1. Jonas Jonasson, *The 100-Year-Old Man Who Climbed out the Window and Disappeared* (New York: Hyperion, 2012). German: *Der Hundertjährige, der aus dem Fenster stieg und verschwand* (Munich: Carl's Books, 2011).

2. Glenda Green, *Love without End: Jesus Speaks* (Sedona, Ariz.: Spirits, 2002). German: *Unendliche Liebe—Jesus spricht* (Burgrain, Germany: Koha, 2014).

3. Green, *Love without End*. German: *Unendliche Liebe—Jesus spricht,* 403 and following.

About the Author

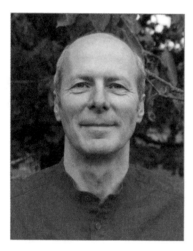

Anton Stucki has always been interested in ideas. First educated in business, he expanded his knowledge by studying physics, biology, mathematics, medicine, and architecture. With this diverse background he began coaching product developers and corporations to help turn their ideas into reality.

In 1998 he founded and became executive partner of MUNDUS GmbH, a company that supports and creates economic platforms for innovative ideas that strive to create harmony between humans and the environment. With a focus on responsible and sustainable thought and action, MUNDUS products encompass the fields of health and healing, prevention, information, awareness, vibration, and healing.

Stucki developed the natural sound transducer known as the Naturschallwandler (NSW) and the MUNDUS method of natural hearing regeneration to help people relearn the basics of hearing and listening through physically correct training. For more information and to view a current list of therapists in Germany, Austria, and Switzerland who use this method, visit the Naturschallwandler website, which can be translated into English using Google, under the tab "traders and therapists."

You can contact the author directly by writing to him at:

Anton Stucki
Mahlsdorfer Str 12
D-14827
Wiesenburg / Reetz
Germany

Index

Page numbers in *italics* indicate illustrations.

accidents, 87–88

acoustics, 29–36

action, 219–21

activities, pleasant, 235

alignment, 145–47, 166

Alzheimer, Alois, 126

Alzheimer's disease, 126

ambient noise, 190–91

amplitude, 33–34

amygdala, 237

anamnesis, 162

anger, 195

anvil, 17, 197

Aristotle, 83

aspects, 16

assumptions, 199–200

athletes, 211

attachment, release of, 255

autism, 119–20, 126

awareness, 5, 222

Bach, Johann Sebastian, 4

balance, 28–29, 57, 68, 96, 196, 198–99, 219–20

barefoot, 135, 162

barriers, breaking down, 227–29

Basic Therapeutic Method, Natural Sound Source

    Phase 1, Part 1, 136–38, *136, 137*

    Phase 1, Part 2, 138–41, *139–141*

    Phase 1, Part 3, 142–45, *142–144*

    Phase 1, Part 4, 147–48

    Phase 1, Part 5, 148–50, *149–50*

    Phase 1, Part 6, 151

    preparation for, 132–35

Basic Therapeutic Method, Natural Sound Transducer

    Phase 1, Part 1, 164–66, *165*

    Phase 1, Part 2, 166–69, *167–69*

    Phase 1, Part 3, 169–73, *170–71*

    Phase 1, Part 4, 174–75

    Phase 1, Part 5, 176–78, *176–77*

    Phase 1, Part 6, 178

    preparation for, 162–64

bats, brain of, 192

beauty, words of, 123–25

beginnings, 106–8

belief, 199–200

Bell, Alexander Graham, 21

Bending Back and Forth, 68–69

bilateral symmetry, 69, 219–20

birds, 30–31, 32

Blindfolded Identification of Sounds
and Their Location, 207–8

blindfolds, 134, 136, 162

blood pressure, 227

blunt trauma, 87–88

body
manifestation of experiences in,
93–94
storing of experiences, 212–14

body awareness, 27

body geometry, 5, 28, 45–46, 100,
184–85, 187–90
aligning, 145–47, *146*, 173–74
documentation templates, *133, 161*

Boltzmann, Ludwig, 222

bone conduction, 18

boundaries, 158, 205

brain, 2–3, 128, 191, 211–12, 214–16,
214

brain stem, 214–16

Breathing Consciously, 102

building, geometry of acoustics,
109–10

burnout, 68

cachexia, 68

caduceus, 219, *220*

calibrate, 220

campanoid, 40, *41,* 49

Cassidy, Eva, 51, 52, 88, 160

Central America, 219

cerebrum, 214, 215

children, 106–7, 126–27, 207, 253–54

China, 219

chiropractors, 100

Chladni, Ernst, 114–15

Chladni figures, 115

chronic pain, 237–238

cilia, 82

clairvoyance, 211

cochlea, *17,* 17–18, 80–81, *81,* 197,
225, 225–26, 241

coercion, 217

communication, 158

companion, explanation for, 135–36,
164

connective tissue, 196

consciousness, 5, 27–28, 59–60, 195,
199–200, 212, 222

control, 198–99, 201

control system, 210–11

conventional medicine, 240–45

cooking as pleasant activity, 235

Corti cells, 82

cosmic octave, 122–23

Cousto, Hans, 122–23

cranial nerve, 215

cybernetics, 64

cymatics, 115–16

danger, 217

dark glasses, 134, 136, 162

deaf people and vibration, 18

death as an adviser of life, 253

debriefing, 151–52, 178–79

decibels, 21–24, *22*

decisions, 216–18, 234

Depardieu, Gerard, 119–20

difficult listening, 24

dilemmas, 101

disappointment, 195

divine proportions, 187–90, *188, 189*

divine quality, 5
dizziness, 101–3
doctors, 241
documentation, 132–33, 160–61
dolphins, 192
do the right thing, 253
downtime, 151, 178–79
dramatic significance, 202, 214
dualism, 219–21
duplicate, 228–29

eardrum, 17, 101, 197, 241
ear protection, 90–91
ears
    disorders of, 96–105
    structure of, 16–18, *16–17,* 197
    world in, 80–83
ease, 254
EEG, 18
electrical signal transmissions,
    126–27
emotional issues of soul related to
    hearing, 126
emotions, 195, 213, 215, 238, 248
Emoto, Masaru, 123–25, *124*
entropy, 222
Epidaurus, theater of, 109–10, *109*
equilibrium, 68, 96
Eustachian tubes, 197
everything flows, 221–24
exercises, directory of, 256–57
    Balance and Control, 198–99
    Bending Back and Forth, 68–69
    Blindfolded Identification of Sounds
        and Their Location, 207–8
    Breathing Consciously, 102
    Flying across a Meadow, 57–58, *58*

Get Up and Sit Down, 212
Hearing Someone from Behind, 64–65
How Well Do I Hear? 41–56, 129–30
Massaging the Feet, 216
Perceiving a Sound with All the
    Senses, 194–95
Playing Hide-and-Seek, 26
Reading Out Loud, 250–51
Reflecting with a Tree, 217–18
Resonance in Movement, 226–27
Training Solo, 230–33
Walking, the Basic Movement of
    Life, 239–40
Walking Straight Ahead, 196–97
Working with a Mirror, 70–76, *71,*
    72–74, 75
experiences, 212–14, 234
exterior factors, 185
eye covers, 134, 136, 162
eyes, 191

fairy tales, 205
faith, 199–200
faucet, water, 42, 129, 131
feelings, 215
field theory, 14
fight, 215
fine motor control, 196
Finkelstein, Arseny, 192
first steps, 106–7
5-pointed star, *188*
flexibility, 239
flight, 215
flow, 221–24
flowers, 122
Flying across a Meadow, 57–58, *58*
follow life, 253–54

forgetfulness, 126–27
forgiveness, 254–55
freedom, 254
freeze, 214–15
frequency, 33–34

Genesis, book of, 79
German Association of the Deaf, 84
Get Up and Sit Down, 212
goals, 235, 247–50
golden ratio, 187–89, *188, 189*
good/evil, 222
gramma, 39, 206
gravity, law of, 4, 31, 185
Greene, Glenda, 252–55

hammer, 197
hara, 57
harmonic intervals, 112
head position, 145–46
healing, 190, 211
hearing
    consciousness and, 59–60
    disorders of, 96–105
    each person can hear, 15–19
    effect of trauma on, 84–86
    keys to change, 234–40
    as learning process, 60–63
    medicine and, 241–42
    memory and, 125–27
    process of, 19–24
    relearning process, 27–29
hearing aids, 43, 51, 132, 159, 240–47
hearing regeneration. *See* Basic
    Therapeutic Method
Hearing Someone from Behind, 64–65
heartbeat, 215

helplessness, 224
hemispheres, 215, 233, 241
Heraclitus, 221
Hermes, 219
Herodotus, 111
hertz vibration patterns, 120–22, *121*
Hilde's story (planes), 155–57
holograms, 39–40, 206–8
holographic hub (brain), 211–12
holos, 206
hot/cold, 222
How Well Do I Hear?, 41–56,
    129–30, 159
Hüther, Gerald, 211
hyperacusis, 3, 103–5, 235, 238, 248

"I am," 5
illness, 87–88
imbalances, 190
information, 241–42
injury, 87–88
integration, 224–27, *225*
intelligence, 211, 254
interior factors, 185
internal order, 210–11
intervention, 224–25
involuntary nervous system, 196
isolation, 94, 95–96, 202, 214

Jenny, Hans, 115–16, *116*
judgment disorders, 126
juggling as pleasant activity, 235
jumps in sound, 148, 175

Kant, Immanuel, 253
Kepler, Johannes, 111–14
kinesthetic, 221

king penguins, 110
knowledge, 219–21, 229–30
Kymatic (Hans Jenny), 116

labyrinth, 80–81, *81*
language, 78
Lauterwasser, Alexander, 120–22
learning, 106–8
legends, 205
Lego blocks, 222–23, *223*
leopard's spots, 120–21, *121*
ligaments, 196
light, 205
light/dark, 222
liquids, 117–19
listener (role of), 131, 135, 186
listening, 15–17, 67–68, 153
listening axis, 192–93
listening field, 42, 63, 66, 96
listening trauma, 93
location, training to rebuild order,
    130–31
logarithmic function, 21, 23
love, 123–25, 206, 222, 252–53
Love Without End, 252–55

magicians, 205
magnets, 186
martial artists, 211
massage as pleasant activity, 235
Massaging the Feet, 216
materials science, 29
math, 220
matter, 221–22
medicine, 240–45
meditation, 207
membranes and cymatics, 116–17

memory, 5, 59, 125–27, 211
mental conflicts, 97
Message of Water, The, 123–25
metaphors, 34
mice, brain of, 192
mimesis, 83–84
mirror neurons, 220–21
misunderstandings, 184–85
monks, 211
monochords, 110–11
motivation, 200, 234
movement, 226–27
"Mozart effect," 67
MUNDUS. *See* Basic Therapeutic
    Method
mundus (defined), 128
muscles, 196
mundus (defined), 128
music, 67, 108–9, 129, 160
myriad, 77–78

natural law, 200
natural order, 123, 201–2
natural sound source. *See* Basic
    Therapeutic Method, Natural
    Sound Source
natural sound transducer. *See*
    Naturschallwandler (NSW)
natural wave radiation, 40–41
nature, 122–23, 207
Naturschallwandler (NSW), 3,
    129, 155–57, 232–33. *See also*
    Training Phase 1—Natural
    Sound Transducer
    initial listening test with, 48–51
    technical implementation of,
    37–41, *38–39, 41*

nausea as a sign, 186
near-death experiences, 211
near/far, 222
negative emotions, 195
negative experiences, 190
neuroplasticity, 236–37
noise, physical overload of, 88–93
nonintervention, 224–25
notes during method, 132, 160–61, *161*
numbers and relationships, 9–10,
    110–11

Old Testament, 10, 120
omnidirectionality, 40
*100-Year-Old Man Who Climbed Out
    the Window and Disappeared,
    The,* 252
order, 201–2, 207, 237
orientation, 19–20
orientation disorders, 126, 207
Ortner, Martin, 243–44
osteopaths, 100
"Over the Rainbow," 51, 52, 88, 160

pain, 108, 195–96, 236, 237
palpitations as a sign, 186
paralysis, 215, 224
partner (role of), 131, 135, 152, 180,
    186
passive attitude, 234
penguins, 110
Perceiving a Sound with All the
    Senses, 194–95
perception, 18–19, 125, 221
perceptual space, 187
perforation, 89
person, 79

personality changes, 126
personal threat, 94–96
phi, 187
physics, 4–5, 29–36
piano keyboard, 111, *111*
Pidgeon, Rebecca, 160
planetary motion, laws of, 112–14,
    112–13, 114
planets, 112–14, *112–13, 114,* 122–23
Playing Hide-and-Seek, 26
pleasant experiences, 235–36
polarities, 222, 224, 225
possibility, 199–200
processing of perception, 5, 28, 184,
    193, 193–94
progress, 233
propagation in all directions, 31
proportions, 187–90
Pythagoras, 110–11

quality of life, 196
questioning, 199–200

rage, 195
rats, brain of, 192
Reading Out Loud, 250–51
receptive, 80
reference point, 63, 65–66, *66*
Reflecting with a Tree, 217–18
regeneration, 12, 13
regulation, 12, 13, 187
relaxation, 229
repetition, 229–30, 237
resistance, 186, 224, 239
resonance, 35, 40, 186
Resonance in Movement, 226–27
responsibility, 201

retreat, 126
rhythm, 226–27
rigidity, 224
Rig Veda, 120
room, 19–20
running water, 42–43, 131

sacred space, 206–7
Schauberger, Viktor, 123
Schwenk, Theodor, 117, *118*
self-healing, 4, 12–13, 108
self-protection, 228
self-regulation, 2–3, 28, 190, 221
seven-note scale, 110–11
shape formation, 114–19
Sheldrake, Rupert, 14
shock, 94, 95–96, 202, 214
shoes, 135, 162, 216, 231, 232
shoulder axis, 145–46
sickness, 195
silence, 207
sine waves, 226
singing, 108–9, 205
skillful nonintervention, 224–25
sleep, 68
snakes as symbol, 219
socks, 135, 162, 231, 232
sorcerers, 205
soul, 5, 126, 222
sound, 31, 35, 63–64, 78–79,
    114–15, 125, 205
sound radiation, 38–39
sounds and spirituality, 108–9
sound sources, 129
sound therapy, 119–120
sound waves, 16–17, 33–35
South Georgia (islands), 110

"Spanish Harlem," (Rebecca Pidgeon),
    160
spatial awareness, 19–20
spatial localization, 5, 28, 190–93
spatial orientation, 128
speech as transformative, 205
speech disorders, 126
spherical sound waves, 33
spirit, 222
spirituality, 108–9, 211
spontaneous healing, 211
stability, 229, 237
standing waves, 122
stirrup, 197
stress, 67–68, 97, 215, 235
structure, 207
sun, 122–23
sweating as a sign, 186
symmetry, 96
symptoms, 86
system, 2

tai chi as pleasant activity, 235
talking as design and creation process,
    205
technology, music and, 160
templates, reproducible, 258
tendons, 196
tension, 188, 190, 196–98, 217, 228
therapeutic listening fields setup,
    42–43, 49–50, 131, 159
therapeutic seat, *42, 49, 50, 134, 141,
    163, 169*
thinking disorders, 126
three central pillars, 184, 187–94
    body geometry and divine
    proportions, 187–90, *186–89*

processing of perception, 193–94, *193*
spatial localization, 190–93
timelines, 249
tinnitus, 27, 94–95, 97–101, 238
Tomatis, Alfred A., 82, 119–20
Torah, 10
training, 24–25, 219–21, 229–30
Training Phase 1—Natural Sound Source
    Part 1, 136–38, *136–37*
    Part 2, 138–41, *139–41*
    Part 3, 142–45, *142–44*
    Part 4, 147–48
    Part 5, 148–50, *149–50*
    Part 6, 151
Training Phase 1—Natural Sound
    Transducer, 158–64
    Part 1, 164–66, *165*
    Part 2, 166–69, *167–69*
    Part 3, 169–73, *170–71*
    Part 4, 174–75
    Part 5, 176–78, *176–77*
    Part 6, 178
Training Phase 2, 229–30
Training Solo, 230–33
trauma, 185–86, 200–4, 224
    breaking down barriers, 227–29
    effect on hearing, 84–86
    make decisions that work, 216–18
    storage in body, 212–14
    types of hearing trauma, 87–93
triggering event, 203–4
trust, 158, 234
turtle's shell, 120, *121*
twists (as sign of blockage), 188, 190
tympanic membrane, 201

universal energy, 219–20

vagus tensor tympani, 197
Vedas, 120
vegetative nervous system, 237–38
vertigo, 101–3
vestibule, 82–83
vibrations, 16–17, 83, 108–9,
    114–15, 122–23, 205
vision, 61, 63, 125
visualization, 235
vitality, regaining, 208–9
voluntary nervous system, 196

walking, 106–7
Walking, the Basic Movement of Life,
    239–40
Walking Straight Ahead, 196–98
walls, breaking down, 227–29
water, 78, 117–19, 123–25, 129
water faucet, 42, 131
wave phenomena in moving medium,
    117–19
whales, 192
whistling, 205
wisdom, 253
witches, 205
words, 205
Working with a Mirror, 70–76, *71–75*
writing as pleasant activity, 235

yin-yang symbol, 219, 225, *225*
yogis, 211

zero pressure, 33, 40